Caring for Patients
from Different Cultures

Caring for Patients
from Different Cultures

Case Studies
from American Hospitals

Geri-Ann Galanti

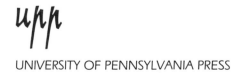

UNIVERSITY OF PENNSYLVANIA PRESS   Philadelphia

Library of Congress Cataloging-in-Publication Data

Galanti, Geri-Ann.
   Caring for patients from different cultures: case studies from
American hospitals / Geri-Ann Galanti.
      p.   cm.
   Includes bibliographical references and index.
   ISBN 0-8122-3065-5 (cloth). — ISBN 0-8122-1344-0 (pbk.)
   1. Transcultural nursing—Case studies.   2. Transcultural medical
care—Case studies.   3. Hospital patients—Medical care—
Psychological aspects—Case studies.   4. Ethnopsychology—Case
studies.   I. Title.
   [DNLM: 1. Anthropology, Cultural.   2. Ethnopsychology.
3. Hospitalization. GN 270 G146c]
RT86.54.G35   1991
610.73—dc20
DNLM/DLC
for Library of Congress   90-13173
                                                              CIP

for my students . . .
who taught me everything I know
and for my husband . . .
who encouraged me to share it

Contents

Preface

The work that resulted in this book began in 1980, when I taught my first medical anthropology class at California State University, Los Angeles. The research continued for a decade while I taught nursing students there, at Chapman College, and, particularly, at the Statewide Nursing Program.

The credit for the book belongs to the thousands of nursing students, who over the years have shared with me the frustration of dealing with the huge ethnic populations in Los Angeles. As a teacher, I was idealistic at first. I thought I could give the students the knowledge they would need to provide ethnically appropriate care. I found, however, that most nurses are overworked and have little time to make adjustments for ethnic differences. They work in the "real world," not an academically idealized version of it. Were my classes of no value, then, beyond mere curiosity?

Fortunately, no. I found I could significantly reduce the nurses' stress by explaining *why* their patients acted as they did. They were not deliberately trying to irritate the staff; they were simply behaving according to their customs. When people ask me what I do, I explain that I teach nurses why their patients are *interesting*, rather than annoying. It makes a difference.

Over the years, I found that the most effective way of making a point is to tell a story. People remember anecdotes much better than they do dry facts and theories. Theories that grow out of stories are much easier to grasp and retain than ones presented in a vacuum. I was fortunate in having a constant source of anecdotes—my students. They were working in the field, observing the actual problems that occur as a result of cultural differences. The cases that one class shared with me, I in turn shared with the next.

It was my husband who eventually suggested that I put these

stories down in a book. The first chapter covers basic theoretical concepts. The rest of the book contains the best of the hundreds of incidents of conflict and misunderstanding that my students experienced. I have tried to give solutions or ways to avoid problems whenever possible, although it is not always possible. In every case, however, I have attempted to explain *why* people acted the way they did. I hope that the book will help readers to see things through the eyes of people from cultures that are different from theirs. For me, that is the greatest contribution anthropology can make to the world.

My only fear is that people of different ethnic groups will read this book and feel they have been presented in a bad light or that the individual in the case described is a poor representative of their ethnic group. Such accusations would not be entirely unjustified. I have chosen cases that created the greatest trouble for the hospital staff, and the individuals involved may not represent the best of their ethnic groups. I have tried to choose examples of behavior that reflect cultural values or customs, even if the behavior is an extreme version. It is my intention to promote understanding, not prejudice. (Troublesome members of my own ethnic group are also well represented here.) I will make a blanket apology at the outset, lest I offend anyone. Truly, no offense is meant.

The book is organized into eight chapters. The first introduces the basic relevant anthropological concepts, and the following six are arranged according to topic: communication, religion and beliefs, family, men and women, birth, and folk medicine. The final chapter is a brief summary. I chose a topical organization, rather than one by ethnic group, both to be in keeping with standard nursing texts and because I felt it was more suitable for making theoretical points. The chapter divisions, however, are somewhat arbitrary. There may be material in one chapter that could just as easily fit into another. Some material did not fit well into any chapter but did not warrant a separate one. Life does not tend to fit into neat categories.

To help readers who might be more comfortable with other organizational schemes, I have constructed an index to the case studies which cross-references each incident in a variety of ways. I hope this will provide greater flexibility for the reader. The first chapter should be read first, but the rest of the book may be read in any order.

I decided to use names for all the patients and hospital staff in the various case studies; it makes the stories more accessible. I tried to use ethnically appropriate names whenever possible. All names are fictitious. If I inadvertently used someone's real name, it was accidental. I used first names for the nurses and last names for the doctors to reflect their usage in practice. For the patients, I used first names for individuals under thirty and last names for those older, simply to provide variety.

The major goal of the book is to help health care professionals recognize the cultural dimensions of problems that occur in hospitals between and among patients, their families, and staff. Obviously, not every possible problem can be documented. There is no easy "recipe" for solving problems; each individual and situation is different. My hope is that this book will give the reader some idea of the range of cultural behaviors and the need to understand people's actions from their own cultural perspective.

The bibliography is intended as a resource guide for those who want to do more research, either out of general interest or to deal with specific problems. It is divided into three subjects: general texts and articles on transcultural nursing and medical anthropology, ethnic groups, and special topics. The list is by no means exhaustive, but it should provide a useful starting point.

Acknowledgments

I want to thank the many people who made this book possible. First, I am grateful to the hundreds of nurses who generously shared with me the cross-cultural misunderstandings they encountered in their work. Next, I am indebted to my parents, Jean and Isaac Galanti, and my brother, Bryan, for so much. Although my father did not live to see this book, he was instrumental in instilling in me the intellectual drive and persistence necessary for such an undertaking. I want to express my appreciation to my professors at UCLA, Robert Edgerton, Allen Johnson, Susan Scrimshaw, and Lowell Sever, for the various roles they played in starting and propelling my career in medical anthropology. The Department of Anthropology at California State University, Los Angeles, hired me to teach my first class in Medical Anthropology. The Statewide Nursing Program had the wisdom to make Culture and Health a required course. I am grateful that both departments have frequently seen fit to assign these courses to me and thus provide me access to the students whose stories lie within. Although I have little experience with editors, I'm sure no one could be more conscientious or encouraging than Patricia Reynolds Smith.

My husband, Don Sutherland, originally conceived of the book. Although he refused to do any of the work, he did live—uncomplainingly—with a mine field of papers all over the floor. Linda Rodgers provided invaluable editing and advice on the original manuscript. Shirley Renz, R.N., M.S.N., and Rich Delingher, M.D., read the manuscript and provided technical advice. I can't adequately express my gratitude to all of them, most especially Don, and for much more than just this book.

It feels wrong to be thanking people and not mention my friends (some of whom are also relatives). They mean everything to me. There are so many people I care about, I am reluctant to mention them by name for fear that, like the flustered Oscar winner, I might leave someone out. They know who they are and how much I care about them. Finally, I want to thank Norman Klein. He knows what for.

Chapter 1
Basic Concepts

If the United States is a melting pot, the cultural stew still has a lot of lumps.

Introduction

What happens when an Iranian doctor and a Filipino nurse treat a Mexican patient? When a Navaho patient calls a medicine man to the hospital? Or when an Anglo nurse refuses to take orders from a Japanese doctor? Generally, the result is confusion and conflict, unless they all have some understanding of cultural differences.

The health care system in the United States has been in a state of crisis for some time. An obvious problem is the cost and apportionment of medical care. A more subtle problem that is beginning to receive attention involves the cultural gap between the medical system and the huge number of ethnic minorities it serves.

The goal of the medical system is to provide optimal care for all patients. In a multiethnic society, this can be accomplished only if the health care providers understand such things as why Asian patients rarely ask for pain medication whereas patients from Mediterranean countries seem to need it for the slightest discomfort, why Middle Eastern patients will not allow a male physician to examine their women, and that coin-rubbing is an Asian form of medical treatment, not a method of child abuse.

This book addresses the cultural differences that create conflicts and misunderstandings and that may result in inferior medical care. First, however, some basic understanding of anthropological principles is required. The remainder of this chapter is devoted to several of the more important concepts. Many will be reviewed in the chapters that follow as well, when the incidents that illustrate the principles are described.

Culture

A basic working definition of culture is that it encompasses beliefs and behaviors that are learned and shared by members of a group.

A man I know removes his shoes when he enters the house. He has indoor shoes and outdoor shoes and will not wear one for the other. Is this a cultural trait or a personal idiosyncrasy? From the information given, it is impossible to tell. One must know his ethnic background. If he were Japanese, it would be a cultural trait. He is not. He is a white Anglo-Saxon Protestant from New York. Thus this trait is a personal idiosyncrasy. For behavior to be cultural, it must be *learned* and *shared* by members of a group. New York WASPs do not make a practice of removing their shoes when entering a house. The Japanese do.

Stereotype versus Generalization

I will be making many generalizations in this book. They should not be mistaken for stereotypes. A stereotype and a generalization may appear similar, but they function very differently. An example is the assumption that Mexicans have large families. If I meet Rosa, a Mexican woman, and I say to myself, Rosa is Mexican; she must have a large family, I am stereotyping her. But if I think Mexicans often have large families; I wonder if Rosa does, I am making a generalization.

A stereotype is an ending point. No attempt is made to learn whether the individual in question fits the statement. A generalization is a beginning point. It indicates common trends, but further information is needed to ascertain whether the statement is appropriate to a particular individual. Generalizations may be inaccurate when applied to specific individuals, but anthropologists do apply generalizations broadly, looking for common patterns, for beliefs and behaviors that are shared by the group. It is important to remember, however, that there are always differences between individuals.

Factors other than innate personality can cause individuals to deviate from the norm for their culture. These factors include the length of time they have spent in the United States, the age at which they came here, their desire to assimilate, whether they live in an ethnic community or an "American" one, whether they came from a rural or urban area, and their level of education. Social and economic class can be even more important than ethnic background. Middle-class Blacks, for example, often have more in common with middle-class Caucasians than with lower-class Blacks.

I have purposely chosen examples of individuals who have not assimilated to a great degree and whose beliefs and behaviors deviate from those expressed in the American health care system. It should not be inferred that all or even most members of these groups will act in the manner described. The ones who are most Westernized do not generally present problems. It is those who adhere to traditional ways that are most likely to, hence their inclusion in this book. It should be remembered, however, that assimilation occurs in unpredictable stages. Individuals may be quite Westernized in some areas but traditional in others.

I frequently make general statements about large groups such as Asians or Hispanics, but they should not be considered a single ethnic group. There are vast differences, for example, between Koreans, Chinese, and Japanese, and between Mexicans, Puerto Ricans, and Peruvians. General statements tend to crosscut the individual groups within the larger one, but obviously differences exist. Members of one Asian group may resent being "lumped" together with members of another Asian group, especially if they are historical enemies. South Americans often look down on Central Americans, who look down on each other. Ethnic pride is strong. Therefore, generalizations about the larger groups may be seen as a way of distinguishing broad geographical groupings from each other while recognizing that there are differences between them. Also, on occasion, the only ethnic identity given for a patient is Asian or Hispanic because more detailed information was not known, but the case illustrated a general point common to most cultures within that group.

Values

Values are the things we hold as important. Just as each individual holds certain values, each culture promotes different ones. American culture (and I use this term loosely because there are literally hundreds of subcultures within the United States) currently values such things as money, freedom, independence, privacy, health and fitness, and physical appearance.

One way to assess a culture's values is to observe how it punishes people. In the United States wrongdoers are punished by being fined (taking away their *money*) or incarcerated (taking away their *freedom*). The Mbuti pygmies of Africa value social support, and they punish people by ignoring them. The kind of health care provided by the

American medical system is often influenced by financial consider-
ations, whereas concern for family, low on the list of "American" values,
influences much patient behavior. Hence conflict may develop between health care providers and patients.

In the United States, *independence* is manifested by the desire to
move away from home as soon as one is financially able. In many
cultures that value family more than independence, adult children
rarely move out before marriage and often not thereafter. The health
care culture also supports the value of independence in its efforts to
teach self-care and in often giving information only to the patient,
excluding other family members.

Privacy is also very important to most Americans, who build fences
to separate their houses from each other. If Americans can afford it,
they provide a separate bedroom for each child. I found a contrasting
situation when I did fieldwork in a remote Guatemalan village. Although land was plentiful and building materials abundant, houses
were built with only one or two bedrooms. Three generations would
often sleep in the same room. It was not that they could not afford
more rooms; they simply did not think of it. They liked being together.
The U.S. health care culture tries to provide privacy for patients by
limiting visiting hours and offering no sleeping accommodations for
visitors. Many non-Anglo patients, however, prefer just the opposite.

Health and fitness are popular movements, particularly on the West
Coast. When reports came out that oat bran lowers cholesterol, several
new oat bran cereals appeared on the market. Quaker Oats sold as it
never had before. People can be seen jogging on most city streets, and
attendance at gyms is high. This obsession with health leads the medical profession to expect patients to comply with suggestions regarding
changes in diet and exercise, assuming that health and fitness is a value
shared by all. It is not. Furthermore, what is considered "healthy"
varies cross-culturally.

Concern for *physical appearance* is manifested at every magazine
stand. There are few women's magazines that do not have articles on
the latest diet, makeup, hairdo, and clothing. The incidence of cos-
metic surgery for both men and women is at a record high. Surgical
techniques are developed to minimize scarring and maintain beauty.
What is considered "beautiful," however, is not the same for every
culture.

Understanding people's values is the key to understanding their
behavior, for our behavior generally reflects our values. A dramatic
example occurred in the early 1980s, when a Japanese ship captain was
bringing a boatload of cars to the United States. There was a disaster at
sea, and the cargo was ruined. The captain had done nothing to cause

the disaster, and he could not have prevented it. If an American ship captain had had a similar experience, the first thing he probably would have done when he reached land was call his insurance agent to see who would pay for the damages. The Japanese captain killed himself.

There is obviously a big difference between calling one's insurance agent and killing oneself. The different reactions are dictated by different values. The hypothetical American captain would probably value *money;* his concern would be for the financial loss. The Japanese captain was concerned with his *honor.* As the captain of the ship, he considered himself responsible for the accident. The loss of the cargo meant the loss of his honor. Without honor, he felt he could not live. Committing ritual suicide was the only way for him to regain his honor.

Values influence our everyday behavior as well. Why are you reading this book? Is it because you value knowledge and hope to learn something? Is it because you are required to read it for a course and you value good grades? If so, are you motivated because good grades will get you a better job, and with a better job you will earn more money, and you value money? Nearly everything we do reflects our values on some level.

All values are not alike, however. There are *real* values, the ones we practice, and *ideal* values, the ones we give lip service to. They do not always overlap. For example, honesty is an ideal American value. To illustrate the importance of honesty, schoolchildren are taught the apocryphal story that George Washington confessed to chopping down a cherry tree. Yet how many people actually submit a tax return that is 100 percent accurate? Or tell a friend that her awful new haircut looks awful? Or, in an overpriced restaurant, admit to having been slightly undercharged? Honesty is an ideal value for most Americans, but it varies in strength as a real value.

World View

The second most important concept for understanding people's behavior is to understand their world view. People's world view consists of their basic assumptions about the nature of reality. These become the foundation for all actions and interpretations. Religion largely defines the world view of people who are devoutly religious. Belief in the existence of God, for example, would be part of their world view. If people believe God confers both health and illness, it may be very difficult to get them to take certain medications or change their health behavior. They would see no point worrying about high blood pressure or germs when moral behavior is the key to good health.

Young children's lies provide insight into their world view and evidence that they have not yet learned their culture's version. For example, a two-year-old boy was playing with his mother's beaded necklace and broke it. She found him on the bed; the beads were all over the room. When she asked him what had happened, he earnestly explained that the necklace suddenly flew apart. He assured her that he had nothing to do with it. He had not yet learned that this is impossible. In his world view, objects *could* suddenly fly apart of their own volition.

Since people's world view consists of their *assumptions* about the nature of reality, they rarely question the veracity of their beliefs. To use an example, the Azande of Central Africa traditionally believed in oracles. Oracles are beings or supernatural forces which can be consulted to reveal information that is otherwise unknowable. They were often used by the Zande to predict the outcome of specific important events such as choosing a new homestead or a wife. The poison oracle was a red powder made from a forest plant and mixed with water to a paste. The liquid was squeezed out of the paste into the beak of a chicken, who was forced to swallow it. Violent spasms usually followed, resulting in the chicken's death or recovery. The outcome signified the oracle's verdict. Explicit ritual instructions had to be followed throughout, and the person administering the poison was required to adhere to several dietary and sexual taboos.

If a Zande had, for example, selected a site for a new home, but wanted to make sure it was a good one, he might consult a poison oracle. After making the proper ritual preparations, he would present the question in a manner that could be answered by yes or no. It was decided beforehand whether the death or recovery of the chicken was an affirmative or negative response.

Suppose recovery signified yes and death no. "Is the site I've selected near the river a good place to build a house?" The poison is fed to the chicken, and the chicken lives. The oracle has spoken. It is a good place to build. The man then proceeds to build his home there. Two weeks after it is completed, there is a tremendous storm and the river overflows, destroying his house. Does this mean the oracle was wrong?

From an outsider's perspective, yes, the oracle was clearly wrong. It was a terrible place to build a house. From the Zande perspective, no. The oracle could not be wrong because one of their basic assumptions about the nature of reality is that oracles are *never* wrong. It would not occur to them to consider the possibility that an oracle could make a mistake. In fact, apparent failures on the part of the oracle's predictions served only to strengthen their beliefs in witchcraft, sorcery, and taboos. If the oracle appeared to be wrong, it was proof that witchcraft was so powerful it could affect even the outcome of the poison oracle.

Or it was evidence that the petitioner neglected to adhere to one of the taboos. A Zande would never conclude that oracles can be wrong on the basis of an inaccurate prediction, any more than a devout Christian would conclude that God does not exist on the basis of the accidental slaughter of innocent children. Rather, the Christian would see it as further proof that "God works in mysterious ways." No matter how much "evidence" is presented to the contrary, people rarely change or even question their world view. Instead, they re-interpret events in a manner consistent with their beliefs.

Voodoo death presents an interesting example of how people interpret events according to their world view. Death by hex has been well documented in many countries, including Haiti, Brazil, Hawaii, New Guinea, and Africa. When autopsies have been done, death is generally found to have been caused by a heart attack, in the absence of heart disease. This phenomenon has attracted the attention of Western scientists and doctors, for in the Western world view it is impossible. Westerners have attempted to explain it as resulting from stress, loss of will to live, and sly poisoning. The knowledge that someone has put a curse on a person may be enough to cause a heart attack; intense shock leads to fear and culminates in death, as Walter Cannon hypothesized in his classic article on the subject. Or a person may psychologically give up after being cursed, feeling the situation is hopeless. Or perhaps the person who placed the curse also slipped lethal poison into the victim's food. Such theories are appealing because they explain the unexplainable within the context of the Western world view. Western medicine understands the physiological mechanisms underlying the stress response. It acknowledges the power of the mind to affect the body via the placebo effect. It also believes in the efficaciousness of poison.

When such discussions arise in my class, I ask the group how many believe their thoughts can harm another person, even if that person has no knowledge of the thoughts. One or two people usually raise their hands. Then I ask how many believe their thoughts or prayers can help heal someone, even if that person does not know about it. Generally, most people raise their hands. When I point out the apparent contradiction in their votes—either their thoughts can affect the health of another person or they cannot, they look uncomfortable. Some will argue (reflecting their world view) that God does the healing when they pray. I respond that if God exists, then does not Satan? If God can act upon their prayers, could not Satan act upon their negative thoughts? An uneasy silence usually follows.

Most cultures believe in the existence of power. Power, like fire, is neither good nor evil, but can be used for both. Fire can provide light and warmth, or it can bring destruction. Power can heal or harm, depending upon the intention and skill of the person using it. Nursing culture tends to believe only in the power of good.

The Westerners' explanations for voodoo death are *etic* explanations. Someone from a culture that believes in voodoo death would explain the death as resulting from the power of the curse. That would be the *emic* explanation. The terms "emic" and "etic," derived from linguistics and rarely used in ordinary life, are extremely important in anthropology. They refer to perspectives. The emic perspective is the insider's perspective, the native's view of his or her own behavior. The etic perspective is that of an outsider. These two simply represent different vantage points, and knowing both helps provide a more complete picture, a fact which caregivers would do well to remember when treating patients from different cultures.

Another aspect of world view involves people's relationship to nature. American culture, for example, believes people can control nature. If the land is dry, they irrigate. If the disease is caused by bacteria, they destroy them. If the heart does not work, they replace it. Other cultures, such as Asian and Native American, see people as a part of nature. They strive to maintain harmony with the earth, and look to the land to provide treatment for disease. Herbal remedies are important in their cultures. Still other cultures, such as Hispanic, believe people have little or no control over natural forces. *Que será, será.* Preventive health care measures are likely to be ignored. They would do no good anyway. What will be, will be. Thus world view can have important implications for health-related behavior.

Ethnocentrism and Cultural Relativism

Two key anthropological concepts are ethnocentrism and cultural relativism. They refer to attitudes. Ethnocentrism is the view that one's culture's way of doing things is the right and natural way. All other ways are inferior, unnatural, perhaps even barbaric. Cultural relativism is the attitude that other ways of doing things are different but equally valid. It tries to understand the behavior in its cultural context. Most humans are ethnocentric. It is natural to think one's own culture's way is best. Anthropologists, however, strive to be culturally relativistic.

If I were to tell most Americans about a group of people in Africa who sometimes kill healthy newborn infants, they would probably take the ethnocentric attitude that these people were barbarians. If I were to explain that they were hunters and gatherers living on the edge of starvation and that if a second child is born too close to the first, chances are about 100 percent that both will die because the mother does not have enough milk to support both, their attitude might change. They still might not condone infanticide, but they might understand it as the only viable choice in a desperate situation. Rather than seeing the Africans as barbarians, they might realize that the people were forced to extreme measures by hopeless circumstances. Their attitude would thus change from being ethnocentric to culturally relativistic.

The Western health care system tends to be ethnocentric because practitioners believe that their approaches to healing are superior to all others. There is a lot we can learn, however, from other cultures. Many modern drugs, including quinine, were derived from plants used by native peoples. Westerners are beginning to acknowledge the effectiveness of acupuncture for certain conditions. The goal of all systems of healing is the same—to help people get well. If all cultures could study each other's techniques with a culturally relativistic perspective, the cause of modern medicine would be greatly advanced.

Several years ago, I interviewed two former members of the Hare Krishna for a research project on cult deprogramming. I was ethnocentrically pleased to find toilet paper in their bathroom, for I had remembered reading that they washed after using the toilet instead. I carelessly remarked to one of them that they must be glad to use toilet paper again. The woman thought for a moment and then responded that she had gotten used to it but that the Hare Krishna way was much cleaner. All toilet paper does is to spread the feces around.

Presented with the emic perspective, I suddenly saw things differently. I went from an attitude of ethnocentrism to cultural relativism in an instant. My aim in writing this book is to help the reader experience that shift in consciousness and be able to see things from another point of view.

Time Orientation

Time orientation, one's focus regarding time, varies in different cultures. No individual or culture will look exclusively to the past, present, or future, but most will tend to emphasize one over the others. Chinese, British, and Austrian cultures have a past orientation. They are traditional and believe in doing things the way they have always been done. Interestingly, in many cases, countries that emphasize the past are ones that were once more powerful than they are now. This may be their way of recognizing and valuing that time in their history. These cultures usually prefer traditional approaches to healing rather than accepting each new procedure or medication that comes out.

Hispanics and Blacks tend to have a present time orientation. This does not mean that they do not recognize the past or the future, but living in the present is more important to them. Their concept of the future may also be different from the Anglo concept. For example, Blacks are more likely to say "I'll see you" than "I'll see you tomorrow." The former implies the future but is not specific. The future arrives in its own time. From this point of view, one cannot be late. Conflict may occur, however, in interactions with white middle-class people, for whom time is very specific. Someone who arrives at 3:15 for a 2:30 appointment is late.

People with a predominantly present time orientation may also be less likely to take preventive health measures. They reason that there is no point taking a pill for hypertension when they feel fine, especially if the pill is expensive and inconveniently causes more frequent urination. They do not look ahead in hope of preventing a stroke or heart attack, or they may feel they will deal with it when it happens. Poverty often forces people into a present time orientation. They are not likely to make plans for the future when they are concerned with surviving today.

Middle-class white American culture tends to be future oriented. That is reflected in the medical system's stress on preventive medicine and enthusiasm for each new medical technique or drug. In contrast to past-oriented cultures, progress and change are highly valued. China is also shifting to a future orientation, as evidenced by the long term plan to reduce the country's population by limiting family size.

Hierarchical versus Egalitarian Cultures

Just as cultures differ in time orientation, they also vary in social structure. American culture is organized according to an egalitarian model. Theoretically, everyone is equal. Status and power are dependent upon an individual's personal qualities rather than age, sex, family, occupation, or any other characteristic. In reality, things may operate differently, but we hold equality as our ideal. Some cultures such as Asian are based on a hierarchical model. Everyone is not equal. Status is based on such characteristics as age, sex, and occupation. Status differences are seen as important, and people of higher status command respect. Social structure, then, can have an important influence on the way people interact, as will be seen in many of the examples given later in this book.

Family of Orientation versus Family of Procreation

During the course of their lives, many people are members of two different family groups—the family they are born into and the one they create through marriage and children. Anthropologists distinguish the two as "family of orientation" and "family of procreation." The family of orientation is the one a person is born into, the one to which one first orients oneself. It includes the individual, parents, brothers and sisters, and any other household members. The family of procreation is the one formed through marrying and procreating. It includes the individual, spouse, and children. Some cultures, particularly those in which the married couple continues to reside with the parents of the bride or groom, emphasize the family of orientation. Other cultures emphasize the family of procreation. Americans tend to set up their own nuclear family households, and that family takes precedence over all others. The result is a differing set of loyalties, as will be discussed in Chapter 4.

Disease Etiology

Most Americans believe that germs cause disease. Not all cultures share that belief, however. Other causes of disease include upset in body balance; soul loss, soul theft, and spirit possession; breach of taboo; and object intrusion. Treatment for diseases resulting from such etiologies must vary to be appropriate to the cause.

Upset in body balance is a notion that appears to have originated in China and spread from there to influence beliefs in Asia, India, Spain, and Latin America. It refers to the belief that a healthy body is in a state of balance. When it gets out of balance, illness results. In Asia, the balance is between yin and yang. All things in the universe are primarily either yin or yang, including diseases, which may result from excess yin, excess yang, deficient yin, or deficient yang. Yin and yang are generally translated as hot (yang) and cold (yin), although these refer to qualities, not temperatures. For example, we perceive chili peppers as hot, even if they have been refrigerated.

The balance between hot and cold can be upset by a number of factors, including an improper balance of foods and strong emotional states. The goal of treatment is to restore balance to the system. This is generally accomplished through the use of foods (for example, cold foods should be eaten to cure a hot illness), herbs, or other treatments. To prevent disease, one should avoid extremes, such as ice water. Diet is exceedingly important. (Dietary staples such as rice are generally thought to be neutral, a fortunate and practical designation.)

Foods that are hot in one culture may be cold in another, so it is difficult to make up a comprehensive list. Patients' beliefs in hot and cold qualities can generally be ascertained only by observing their behavior. If they refuse certain foods or medications it may be that an illness they perceive as hot is being treated with a hot food or medication. Offering other foods or liquids to take with the pill to "neutralize" it may solve the problem. If they will not take the pill with ice water, they might take it with hot tea, orange juice, or hot chocolate.

Although the importance of maintaining a balance between hot and cold is not recognized in Western medicine, there is a growing recognition that stress plays an important role in affecting the immune system's ability to fight disease. Stress represents a kind of imbalance. Recent studies indicate that a person's emotional state may also have a significant influence on the immune system. Thus, though the words we use are different, body balance is a notion to which we should be able to relate.

Paradoxically, China is moving away from traditional medicine in favor of Western medicine, while there is increasing interest in the United States in traditional Chinese healing practices. When I asked several Chinese nurses how they integrate the concept of yin and yang with germ theory, they explained that when yin and yang are out of balance, germs can cause disease. This is nearly identical to the Western notion of the relationship between stress and disease.

Soul loss, along with related *soul theft,* is another category of disease etiology. The concept is self-explanatory. The soul has either left the body on its own or been stolen, leaving the body in a weakened and ill state. The goal of treatment is to return the soul to the body. It usually requires a specialist, such as a shaman, who can "leave" his own body to search for and return the missing soul. Although Western medicine lacks a similar etiological category, catatonic schizophrenics can be described metaphorically as bodies with "no one home."

Spirit possession involves the taking over of the victim's body by a spirit being. The victim usually acts in ways that are inappropriate for him or her. (In some cultures, this may give the victim a form of power. It is generally the poor, the oppressed, and minorities who become "possessed." For example, in Ethiopia, women may become possessed by powerful "Zar" spirits. When this occurs, their husbands must treat them with unaccustomed kindness and respect, for they are no longer dealing with their wives but with powerful Zars. The negative side of possession by a Zar is that the woman is thought to be crazy and must seek help through a Zar cult.) Exorcism is the treatment for spirit possession.

The next etiological category is *breach of taboo,* which means doing something forbidden, whether it is eating food cooked by a menstruating woman, speaking directly to one's mother-in-law, or, among some Christian sects, having extramarital or homosexual relations. Disease is the punishment meted out by a supernatural force such as God. Treatment involves penance and atonement.

The final major category is *object intrusion*. It refers to the condition in which a magical foreign object enters the body and causes the individual to become ill. Treatment involves removing the object. In most cases, a shaman will suck it out from the afflicted part of the patient's body. The shaman then produces the offending object. Upon analysis, the object often turns out to be bits of hair, animal parts, teeth, or plant material, mixed with blood from the shaman's mouth. One shaman, accused by an anthropologist of practicing legerdemain, freely admitted to secreting the object in his mouth prior to sucking it out of the patient's body. He explained that the *real* object he removed was invisible, but that it was important for the patient to see something tangible, so he practiced a bit of sleight of hand (or mouth) for the patient's psychological benefit.

Two important points should be made regarding disease etiology. First, the treatment must be appropriate to the cause. If germs cause disease, kill the germs. If the body is out of balance, restore balance. If the soul is gone, retrieve it. If a spirit has taken over the body, exorcise it. If a rule has been violated, do penance. If an object has entered the body, remove it. All these remedies are perfectly logical. Whether these etiologies are the true causes of the disease is irrelevant. A patient who believes he or she is ill because of soul loss will not be cured by any amount of antibiotics. The mind is very powerful, as the placebo effect demonstrates. The patient's beliefs, as well as body, must be treated. Many Americans feel they have not been treated properly if they do not receive an antibiotic for a virus, even though antibiotics are effective only against bacteria. Psychologically, they need the pill to get well.

Second, we must not let our ethnocentrism blind us to the merits in the beliefs of other cultures. They may be right. It is easy to look down on other systems, citing science to support Western medical beliefs. But *all* medical systems are based on observed cause-and-effect relationships. The major difference with the scientific approach is that science is falsifiable. A scientific hypothesis can be proven wrong. The beliefs of other systems cannot.

At the level of the individual, however, Americans demand no more proof than do people of any culture. Most believe germs cause disease because their mothers told them so. Few have ever actually seen a germ, and fewer demand to see proof of a virus or bacteria at work. The experts have done that, and their word, along with our mothers', is enough. The same is true in other cultures. People believe disease is caused by spirit possession or object intrusion because their mothers and cultural experts told them so. They have seen people become ill when that happens and get well when treated. What further proof is necessary?

Cultural Customs

It can be argued that most cultural practices originate for very practical reasons. People, however, do not always act in a practical manner if the benefit to them is not obvious and immediate. They may need a "higher" purpose. Ideological injunctions are much more likely to be followed, as anthropologist Marvin Harris, a leading proponent of the cultural materialism approach, points out.

For example, the Hindu prohibition against killing cows may seem bizarre in a country where most people are starving, but it has a practical basis. Most cows are malnourished and if slaughtered would provide very little food. Living, however, cows are good substitutes for tractors. Their dung provides fertilizer, fuel for cooking, and, mixed with water, makes an excellent household flooring material. Far more use is made of living cows than could ever be gained from dead ones. Hungry individuals, however, might look at a cow and see dinner. Forgetting the animal's other practical uses, they might kill and eat it. But if the animal is made sacred, religious ideology will prevent such killing.

Circumstances sometimes change, obliterating the practical need for a custom. Ideology, however, is enduring and soon becomes tradition. Although many cultural and religious traditions no longer have any practical value, they have an important psychological one—they provide a sense of identity and belonging. They serve as a strong reminder that the individual is not like everyone else; he or she belongs to a special group. Abstaining from meat when everyone else is having hamburgers reminds the Hindu that he is Hindu. Walking to temple instead of driving on the Sabbath reminds the Jew that she is Jewish. In fact, the more difficult or impractical the custom, the stronger the reminder of ethnic or religious identity. Thus, the benefits of adhering to seemingly outmoded customs can be enormous in a country like the United States, where feelings of isolation and anomie may be strong.

Chapter 2
Communication and Time Orientation

Miscommunication is a frequent problem in hospitals. The most obvious case is when the patient and the hospital personnel do not speak the same language. Interpreters are not always available. When they are, vocabulary may be insufficient. But these problems are obvious. There are more subtle ones that result from cultural differences in verbal and nonverbal communication styles and patterns. This chapter will explore these problems in communication as well as another subtle but provocative source of difficulty—cultural differences in time orientation. Patients and staff members may operate on different "time clocks," causing confusion and resentment for all parties.

The Interpreter

A Hispanic woman, Graciela Garcia, had to sign an informed consent form for a hysterectomy. Her bilingual son served as the interpreter. When he described the procedure to his mother, he appeared to be translating accurately and indicating the appropriate body parts. His mother signed willingly. The next day, however, when she learned that her uterus had been removed and that she could no longer bear children, she became very angry and threatened to sue the hospital. What went wrong?

Because it is inappropriate for a Hispanic male to discuss her private parts with his mother, the embarrassed son explained that a tumor would be removed from her abdomen and pointed to that general area. When Mrs. Garcia learned that her uterus had been removed, she was quite angry and upset because a Hispanic woman's status is derived in large part from the number of children she produces.

The lesson here is that even speaking the same language is not always sufficient. Cultural rules often dictate who can discuss what with whom. In general, it is best to use a same-sex interpreter when translating matters of a private or sexual nature.

Similarly, the husband is not always the best choice for an interpreter in labor and delivery. The answer to the standard question, "How many times have you been pregnant?" may contain secret abortions or even births the woman has kept hidden from her spouse. Honest answers regarding sexual issues are rarely obtained by using family members as interpreters.

Eye Contact

2 Ellen was trying to teach her Navaho patient, Jim Nez, how to live with his newly diagnosed diabetes. She soon became extremely frustrated because she felt she was not getting through to him. He asked very few questions and never met her eyes. She reasoned from this that he was uninterested and therefore not listening to her.

Rather than signaling disinterest, however, Mr. Nez's behavior demonstrated a respect for the nurse's authority. The Navaho value silence. A person who interrupts while someone is speaking is perceived as immature. Most Americans are uncomfortable with silences and tend to fill them with words, making "small" talk. The Navaho use silence to formulate their thoughts. Words should have significance. An anthropologist doing fieldwork among the Navaho commented that it took her a long time to get used to talking with them. She would ask a question and get no response. She assumed they had not heard or understood her. She was wrong. They were trying to give her the most complete answer possible, and that took consideration. Eventually, she became comfortable with long pauses in conversation.

Mr. Nez's lack of eye contact probably reflected the Navaho belief that the eyes are the window to the soul. To make direct eye contact is disrespectful and can endanger the spirits of both parties. Thus his lack of eye contact actually displayed his concern.

A former student said she automatically rejected job applicants who did not make eye contact on the basis that they could not be trusted. In fact, there may be good cultural reasons why eye contact is purposely avoided.

Many Asians consider it disrespectful to look someone directly in the eye, especially if that person is in a superior position. Most Asian cultures are hierarchical; men are considered superior to women, parents to children, teachers to students, doctors to nurses, and so forth. Looking someone directly in the eye implies equality. An Asian patient may avoid eye contact out of respect for the "superior status" of the doctor or nurse, rather than for reasons of disinterest or dishonesty.

Many Middle Easterners regard direct eye contact between a man and a woman as a sexual invitation. Female doctors or nurses dealing with Middle Eastern men must be aware that their eye contact may be interpreted not as directness but as an invitation of a sexual nature. In general, eye contact should be avoided with Middle Easterners of the opposite sex. Medical personnel should be aware of the meaning of eye contact in their patients' culture and make sure the appropriate communication is both transmitted and received.

Idioms

Idioms or other nonliteral expressions can also create misunderstanding. A Chinese-born physician called the night nurse one evening to check on a patient scheduled for surgery the next day. The nurse advised the physician that she noticed a new hesitancy in the patient's attitude. "To tell you the truth, doctor, I think Mrs. Colby is getting cold feet." The physician was not familiar with this idiom, suspected circulation problems, and ordered vascular tests. 3

A nervous patient jokingly asked his surgeon if he were going to "kick the bucket." The Korean physician, wanting to reassure the patient that his upcoming surgery would be successful, responded affably, "Oh, yes, you are definitely going to kick the bucket!" The patient was not reassured. 4

Non-native English speakers may sometimes assign more meaning to a term than is intended. An Anglo nurse was in the habit of helping out nurses' aides when her own work was done. All of the aides but one accepted Sylvia's assistance gratefully. When Sylvia offered to help Celina, a Filipino aide, with the difficult care of her quadriplegic and stroke patients, she declined. Sylvia responded, "Don't be silly! It's crazy to do this alone. You could get a bad back." Celina took the words "silly" and "crazy" literally to mean that Sylvia thought she was mentally ill, a condition that is highly stigmatized in Filipino culture. No wonder she was insulted. Celina also interpreted the original offer of help to mean that Sylvia thought she was slow and incompetent. Her "amor propio" (self-esteem) had been wounded. 5

Sylvia learned of Celina's reaction from another Filipino aide. Celina had not said anything directly to Sylvia because she wanted to avoid conflict and show respect for authority—important values in the Filipino culture. The next time Sylvia saw Celina, she apologized, saying that she had not understood how Celina felt. Celina explained that she had been raised with certain ideas and was having trouble adjusting to American ways. For example, Filipino nurses feel they have failed if they do not complete all their work on an eight-hour shift. American nurses will simply tell those on the next shift that they were very busy and could not finish everything. By the end of their discussion, Celina and Sylvia came to an understanding and never had any more problems. It is important to realize that words and actions can carry greater significance than we might intend.

Another English

Language problems can also occur among native English speakers. In England, South Africa, and Australia, the word "fanny" is a derogatory term referring to a woman's vagina. Imagine the shock and horror of a British woman—or the confusion of a British man—when told to prepare for a shot in the fanny. (A South African nurse was appalled when an American aerobics instructor called out to her class, "Tighten your fanny, shake your fanny!") Similarly, birth control instruction to speakers of the "Queen's English" could be confusing if the instructor referred to a condom as a "rubber." Erasers are not a very effective means of preventing pregnancy.

"Boy"

6   Certain words have negative and inflammatory associations when used by the wrong people. Lavelle, who is Black, was the primary nurse for four sixteen-year-old Black gang members. She had developed a good relationship with them and treated them like her own children. When one got out of line, she would simply say, "Boy, keep your mouth shut and go somewhere and sit down." They usually complied.

One day, Susan, an Anglo nurse, tried the same tactic with one of them. It was time for Earl to go to physical therapy, but he was giving Susan a hard time. She assumed from his smile that he was joking. Finally, she tried Lavelle's approach. "Come on, boy," she said. "I'm not kidding with you. You have to go to therapy."

Earl flew into a rage and started swearing at Susan. Lavelle had to help calm him down. Susan was confused. He had never responded that way to Lavelle. She had not considered that the term "boy" is inoffensive when used by one Black person speaking to another but is highly insulting when used by Caucasians because of its origins among slaveowners.

7   Colleen, an Anglo nurse from Canada, learned the meaning of

"boy" the hard way. Her first job when she moved to the United States was at an inner city hospital. The cafeteria was crowded the first day she was there, but she found an empty place across from two Black men. She went over to them and asked very sweetly, "Do you boys mind if I sit down here?" One answered her by picking up his plate of food and throwing it at her.

Most people would agree that he overreacted, but his response is understandable in the context of race relations in this country. The misunderstanding occurred because Canada has not had the same racial problems as the United States, and in the part of the country Colleen was from, adult men and women commonly refer to each other as boys and girls. No insult is meant or taken. Once someone explained the reason for the man's reaction to Colleen, she did not make that mistake again.

Many people know that "boy" is highly insulting to a Black man, but few are aware that the term "gal" has similar connotations for many Black women. Black slave women were called "gals," which explains why several Anglo nurses reported receiving cold and hostile glares from Black nurses whom they innocently referred to as "gals."

First Names

Blacks' sensitivity to perceived slights to their dignity is not surprising given their history in this country. It is therefore especially important to show them respect. Mary Washington, an elderly Black woman, was in the recovery room after surgery. To assess her condition, Cheryl, her nurse, spoke her name, "Mary." The patient slowly opened her eyes and turned her head but made no further sign of acknowledgment. Cheryl became concerned because most patients responded readily and clearly at this point. Shortly afterward Cheryl called the woman Mrs. Washington. She then became alert, pleasant, and cooperative. She had perceived the use of her first name as a lack of respect and a form of racism.

Americans tend to refer to each other by their first names. It is considered a sign of friendliness and equality. To use a first name for anyone other than a close friend, however, is both inappropriate and discourteous in most cultures, including European. In nineteenth-century English novels, even teenage girls referred to each other as Miss —— until they had been friends for at least a year. Hospital personnel should refer to all adult patients as Mr., Miss, Ms., or Mrs., unless instructed otherwise.

8

Values and "Yes"

9   Cultural values can also create communication problems. Jackie, an Anglo nurse, was explaining the harmful side effects of the medication Adela Samillan, a Filipino patient, was to take at home after her discharge. Although Mrs. Samillan spoke some English, her husband, who was more fluent, served as interpreter. Throughout Jackie's explanation, the Samillans nodded in agreement and understanding and laughed nervously. When Jackie verbally tested them on the information, however, it was apparent that they understood very little. What had happened?

Dignity and self-esteem are extremely important for most Asians. Had the Samillans indicated that they did not understand Jackie's instructions, they would have lost their self-esteem for not understanding or they would have caused Jackie to lose hers for not explaining the material well enough. By pretending to understand, Mr. and Mrs. Samillan felt they were preserving everyone's dignity.

Jackie's first clue should have been their nervous laughter. Asians usually manifest discomfort and embarrassment by giggling. Once Jackie realized they had not understood the material, she went over it until they were able to explain it back to her. It is important not to take smiles and nods of agreement for understanding when dealing with Asian patients. They should be asked to demonstrate their understanding.

10   The above incident sheds light on a perplexing situation that occurred when Marsha, an Anglo nurse, attempted to assess the knowledge and technical skills of the critical care nurses in her hospital. Most were from China, Laos, Korea, Vietnam, and the Philippines. The first phase of testing involved a written exam focusing on general principles. Confusion reigned, and the scores were low. Thinking the problem lay in the language of the test, Marsha rewrote the exam. In the new version, the nurses had only to answer yes or no to questions about their knowledge of a specific procedure (e.g., "I understand the principles of hemodynamic monitoring"). Over 90 percent of the questions received a "yes" response. Disturbed by the contradictory results of the two tests, Marsha interviewed several of the test-takers, asking open-ended questions which required them to demonstrate their knowledge. Although their English was proficient, many were unable to answer correctly. Why did they say they understood procedures and principles they clearly did not?

As with the previous case, the Asian nurses were too embarrassed to admit they did not know something. Education is highly valued, and a lack of knowledge indicates a lack of education. The result is a loss of self-esteem. The moral is the same—do not take a "yes" answer at face value.

A third incident involved Linh Lee, a sixty-four-year-old Chinese woman hospitalized for an acute evolving heart attack. At discharge, her physician suggested that she come back in two weeks for a follow-up examination. She agreed to do so, but never returned. It is likely that she never intended to do so but agreed because he was an authority figure. Chinese are taught to value accommodation. Rather than refuse to the physician's face and cause him dishonor, Mrs. Lee agreed. She simply did not follow through, sparing everyone embarrassment. When Nancy, her Chinese-American nurse, saw her in Chinatown several weeks later, Mrs. Lee was very cordial and said she was feeling fine.

The cases described above involved the use of the word "yes" to avoid the embarrassment of saying no. There is another occasion in which "yes" may be used inappropriately (from the American perspective), for reasons of grammar. According to common English usage, if someone were asked, "Haven't you eaten yet today?" and they had not eaten, they would answer, "No." According to Asian grammar, the accurate response would be "Yes," as in "Yes, it is a true statement that I have not yet eaten today." The English speaker would be misled by the Asian patient's affirmative response, thinking that person had already eaten when he or she had not. To reduce possible confusion, it is generally best to avoid sentences with negatives.

Pronouns

Different languages have characteristics that are not directly translatable, as anyone who has struggled with the task of remembering the gender of inanimate objects in French or Spanish knows well. English poses a similar problem for many Asians.

Mieko, a Japanese nurse, was assigned to care for six patients, two male and four female. During report, she consistently referred to the female patients as "he." Her supervisor interrupted to point out that there were no male patients in the bed numbers she mentioned. Mieko acknowledged that fact and continued in the same manner. The supervisor became confused. Had four transsexuals slipped in?

The explanation is simple. Many Asian languages lack pronouns that reflect sex; "he" and "she" do not exist. Thus Asians have no model for using "he" or "she" and often mix them up, confusing everyone else in the process. Knowledge of this characteristic of the language can cut down on the confusion.

Gestures

13   Nonverbal communication can be equally problematical. An Anglo patient named Jon Smith called out to Maria, a Filipino nurse: "Nurse, nurse." Maria came to Mr. Smith's door and politely asked, "May I help you?" Mr. Smith beckoned for her to come closer by motioning with his right index finger. Maria remained where she was and responded in an angry voice, "What do you want?"

Mr. Smith was confused. Why had Maria's manner suddenly changed? The problem was that the innocent "come here" gesture is used in the Philippines only to call animals, and in a sense Mr. Smith had called Maria a dog. To summon a person, Filipinos motion with the whole hand, palm in, fingers up. Unfortunately, many Americans are confused as to whether this gesture means "come here" or "go away."

Problems such as this can best be handled through in-service education classes. If hospital personnel from other cultures are taught the different meanings of gestures, they might not take offense. Maria might have responded to Mr. Smith's request and then politely explained how she felt about the gesture. Mr. Smith would have learned something important about cross-cultural communication and probably refrained from using that gesture with a Filipino again.

Other seemingly innocuous gestures that can create misunderstandings include the "okay" sign (thumb and index fingers together in a circle, other fingers straight up), the "thumbs-up" sign, and the "V" made with the index and middle fingers (used to signify either peace or victory). In Brazil, the "okay" sign is a crude sexual invitation. "Thumbs-up" in Iran and the "V," held palm in, in South Africa are insulting gestures similar to the raised middle finger in U.S. culture.

Demeanor

14   A twenty-seven-year-old Mexican-American named Alfredo Gomez was in traction with multiple fractures following a car accident. He whined continuously and incessantly summoned Helga, his German nurse, with the call light. Helga became very frustrated and angry with him and consequently adopted a stern and direct attitude. Alfredo's behavior changed only when his wife and sister arrived and gave him their full attention. They anticipated his every need, straightening his pillow and moistening his lips. Following their lead, Helga spoke more slowly and warmly to Alfredo, letting him know she understood what a frightening experience he had had. She also did what she could to

make him more comfortable before he asked. As a result, he quickly became less dependent and did not use the call light so frequently.

Why did Helga's change in behavior have this positive effect on him? Helga had been raised to be strong and stoic when ill and thus had little tolerance for Alfredo's whining and demanding behavior. She treated him unemotionally, in the proper German manner. Mexicans, in contrast, are far more emotionally expressive. They expect to be pampered when ill; it is one way the family shows love and concern. Alfredo was feeling alone, frightened, and unloved because he was not receiving the care and attention he expected. He became even more needy. Once he was treated the way he expected to be, his anxiety and thus his neediness were lessened.

Another difficult patient was a twenty-five-year-old upper-class   15
Iranian named Hamid Sadeghi. He was very uncooperative and refused to do anything for himself. He would ring for the nurses and demand, "You get here right now and do this." He would not, however, accept anything he had not specifically requested, including lunch trays and medication. He posted a sign on his door that read, "Do not enter without knocking, including the nurses." His attitude caused a great deal of resentment among the nurses. Why did he treat them this way?

When asked, Hamid responded, "This is the way it is done." Finally, one of the nurses who had an Iranian brother-in-law recognized the behavior and explained. Traditionally, Iranian men are dominant over Iranian women. They *give* orders to women, not take them. Furthermore, as a member of the upper class, Hamid was probably used to giving orders to servants. He was not purposely being difficult but merely acting in his customary manner.

Nursing is a low-level position in the Middle East because the job requires a woman to violate the laws of the Koran—she must both look at and touch the bodies of naked male strangers. The Koran stipulates extreme sexual segregation, primarily to protect the purity of women. Middle Eastern men may thus have little respect for the female nurse who trespasses their sacred laws in the performance of her duties. It is no wonder that Saudi Arabians pay huge salaries to foreign nurses; it is difficult to attract many Saudi women to the profession.

There was no happy resolution to Hamid's situation. Some of the nurses complied with his demands, some refused to care for him. All resented him. Once the nurses understood the reason for his behavior, they tried to discuss it with him. Their efforts went unrewarded, however, because Hamid was unwilling to accept American culture and they were unwilling to adapt themselves to his. The doctor tried to intervene, but Hamid would not budge. "I will treat the nurses as women should be treated," he maintained.

The nurses eventually pressured the doctor to discharge the patient because no one wanted to care for him. The doctor felt an early discharge would not endanger him, and Hamid was quite willing to leave. The incident did nothing to promote cross-cultural communication. Hamid's behavior toward the nurses was extreme, but it was based on Middle Eastern sex roles. A better solution would have been to assign a male nurse to his case.

Expression of Pain

16 David Stein, a twenty-two-year-old Jewish patient suffering from fractured ribs following an auto accident, was both demanding and expressive. He made no effort to do anything for himself. David continually pushed the call light to have someone come straighten his covers or hand him the urinal, even though it was within easy reach. He brushed his teeth only when June, his nurse, steadfastly insisted. When he was turned over, stuck for lab work, or had his intravenous line restarted, he screamed so loudly that June was afraid people would think he was being tortured. When his mother came to visit, she hovered over him and acted solicitous.

A classic study done in a New York hospital in the early 1950s sheds some light on David's behavior. Mark Zborowski's project focused on three groups: Jews, Italians, and "Old Americans" (WASPs). These groups were selected because Jews and Italians had a reputation for exaggerating their pain, whereas the behavior of Old Americans was consistent with the values of the medical system; they were stoic and undemanding.

Although Jews and Italians reacted similarly to pain—loudly—they did so for different reasons. The Italians complained because the pain hurt. Pain medication usually satisfied them. This remedy was rarely effective with Jewish patients, however. In addition to everything else, they would then worry about becoming addicted. Their primary concern was not the pain sensation but the meaning and significance of the pain. How would it affect them and their families?

Zborowski observed that Jews and Italians have a similar socialization process. Children are warned to avoid injury, colds, and fights. Crying elicits sympathy, concern, and aid. The more they complain, the more attention and sympathy they receive. In many Jewish families, even a sneeze is seen as illness, thus predisposing children to become anxious about the meaning and significance of any symptoms. Jewish and Italian children are praised for avoiding physical injury and reprimanded for ignoring bad weather, drafts, or playing rough games.

In contrast, Old American children are encouraged to participate in sports. Boys are taught to "take pain like a man" rather than "cry like a sissy" when injured. The body is seen as a machine, which, when not working (that is, when ill or injured) should be taken to a specialist (a doctor) and treated with as little fuss as possible.

Given their upbringings, it should not be surprising that adult Jews and Italians complain and desire attention when ill, while WASPs tend to be "easy" patients. When they are ill, most people revert to childhood behavior, even if the desired results are not forthcoming. If, like the Jewish patient described earlier, they were rewarded for complaining as children, they will complain as adults. If they were taught to lie quietly and not make a fuss, they will probably do the same when they grow up.

Most nurses find it difficult to care for patients like David, whose behavior, like Hamid's, was an extreme version of his culture. Nurses expect stoicism and compliance and do not get it. They thus tend to do as little as possible, and a new nurse is assigned to such patients each day. There are no easy solutions; extreme patience and understanding are required.

Stoicism

In contrast, some patients tolerate even the most severe pain with little   17
more than a clenched jaw and frequently will refuse pain medication. Osito Seisay, a Nigerian farmer who had been injured by a charging bull, was in the United States for arthro-microscopic knee surgery. His nurse waited for him to request pain medication, but he never did. Mr. Seisay was Muslim, and he offered his pain to Allah in thanks for the good fortune of being allowed such specialized surgery.

Asian patients are also known for remaining stoic while in pain.   18
Horace Ling, a sixty-eight-year-old Chinese patient with second-degree burns, continually refused pain medication, despite clinical signs of severe pain. His refusal exacerbated an underlying cardio-vascular problem and resulted in dangerously high blood pressure. His physician, Dr. Stevens, tried to lower the patient's blood pressure through pain medication, but Mr. Ling, practicing traditional stoicism, refused to accept it. Mr. Ling's family supported his wishes, and the nurses felt they too had to respect his rights. Dr. Stevens became angry with the nurses for supporting Mr. Ling's position. Although the medical staff talked to Mr. Ling several times about the need for pain medication, his response was always the same: "No thank you." Some

of the doctors suggested that the nurses "slip some morphine" into Mr. Ling's intravenous line without telling him, but they refused. They were afraid that his relatives, who were always around, would notice.

The staff finally called in a Chinese interpreter to explain the importance of taking pain medication. This act had an unexpectedly negative result. Not only did Mr. Ling continue to refuse medication, but he became upset because the staff thought he was "dumb." Why else would they have sent for an interpreter when he had understood everything perfectly? He simply did not want any pain medication.

The situation resolved itself a week later when Mr. Ling died. Death resulted from secondary complications of the burns, primarily infections. Cardiovascular complications, Dr. Stevens's major concern, did not play a part.

19   Vickie, a research nurse dispensing experimental analgesics, noted that an elderly Filipino patient named Fernando Abatay had not received any pain medication following his shoulder repair. When she asked him how much pain he was experiencing, he replied, "A lot." Vickie then questioned why he had not taken any medication. Mr. Abatay explained, "No one asked me if I wanted a shot and I didn't want to bother the nurses." The regular nurses assigned to him claimed that they could not tell he was in pain, and because he did not request any pain medication, they saw no need to give him any.

Mr. Abatay's behavior can be explained in part by the Filipino concept of *Bahala na* (God's will). Filipinos may appear stoic because they believe pain is the will of God and thus God will give them the strength to bear it. Besides, one cannot change it. This attitude is reminiscent of the fatalistic Hispanic concept *Que será, será.* A second explanation relates to Filipinos' respect for authority. Mr. Abatay did not want to bother the nurses. A professional's time is valuable, and unless one's problem is very serious, it is better left unmentioned.

20   Similarly, a middle-aged Chinese patient named Patrick Chang refused pain medication following cataract surgery. When asked, he replied that his discomfort was bearable and he could survive without any medication. Later, however, the nurse found him restless and uncomfortable. Again, she offered pain medication. Again he refused, explaining that her responsibilities at the hospital were far more important than his immediate comfort and he did not want to impose on her. Only after she firmly insisted that a patient's comfort was one of her most important responsibilities did Mr. Chang finally agree to take the medication.

His attitude is very different from that of most American patients. The Chinese, however, are taught self-restraint. Assertive and individualistic people are considered crude and poorly socialized. The needs of the group are more important than those of the individual. Incon-spicuousness is highly valued and in recent history has proved neces-sary for survival. It is best not to call attention to oneself.

One other factor that may be involved in Asians' refusal of pain medication is courtesy. They generally consider it impolite to accept something the first time it is offered. Several nurses from mainland China said they often went hungry during the first few weeks of their stay in the United States. Whenever someone asked them if they wanted something to eat, they politely refused, awaiting a second offer. It rarely came. They soon learned that in America, if one does not accept something the first time, there may be no second chance. Hospi-tal nurses are so busy that they seldom offer something more than once. They should be aware of Asian rules of etiquette when offering pain medication, food, back rubs, or other services.

The safest approach for the health care professional is to antici-pate the needs of an Asian patient for pain medication without waiting for requests. If patients are told that their doctor ordered the medica-tion, they will be less likely to refuse on the grounds of courtesy. Asians tend to respect the authority of the physician. But if patients continue to refuse medication, their wishes should be respected.

One case involving cultural differences in expressing pain had a   21
tragic ending. The Irish mother-in-law of one of my nursing students was in the hospital. She was scheduled for surgery at the end of the week. Her family became very concerned when she suddenly started complaining of pain. They knew Mrs. Carroll was typically Irish in her stoicism. They spoke to her doctor, who was from India. He was not worried. In his country, women were usually vocal when in pain. He ignored their requests that the surgery be done sooner, thinking it unnecessary.

When he finally did operate, he discovered that Mrs. Carroll's condition had progressed to the point that she could not be saved. It is possible that if he had recognized her expressions of pain as a sign that something was very wrong and had operated sooner, she might have lived.

Refusal to Talk

A nurse experienced great difficulty in obtaining a health history from   22
a young Gypsy woman. The patient's mother-in-law insisted upon accompanying her to the examining room. The nurse assumed she wanted to act as an interpreter, but her English skills were no better than her daughter-in-law's. The patient's reply to every question was the same: "I don't know." She probably knew many of the answers but

was respecting a cultural prohibition against giving too much information to Gaje (non-Gypsies). The patient's mother-in-law may have been there in part to protect her and in part to make sure she did not reveal too much.

23   Another situation involved a twenty-five-year-old Laotian refugee named Thongsouk Vongkhamkaew, who was being treated for stomach cancer. Although her English was proficient, she did not appear to have a full understanding of her disease and the treatments and life changes necessary for coping with it. Greg, a staff social worker, decided to arrange for a translator. When the nurse introduced Greg to Thongsouk so he could explain his plan, she appeared very nervous. She would not talk with him except to repeat, "Everything is okay."

Thongsouk's fear and refusal to talk stemmed from her mistaken belief that Greg was with the military or government. After many decades of war, Laotians tend to distrust strangers. The patient might have feared that anything she said would have repercussions for her family still in Laos and Thailand. She did not understand the role of the social worker. There is no equivalent in Laos, where family and friends provide assistance and support, and hospitals are for medicine. She might have responded better if one of the doctors or nurses, whose role she understood and accepted, had talked with her instead.

Privacy and Personal Matters

24   A fifty-five-year-old Mexican-American woman named Maria Ibañez was admitted to the coronary care unit with chest pain. She appeared withdrawn and was crying. When asked what was wrong, she shook her head and replied, "Nothing." She gave brief answers to Dr. Mandel, the physician who took her family history, but offered no additional information. Her crying continued even after her chest pain ceased, and Dr. Mandel asked why she was depressed. Still she did not answer.

Eventually Mrs. Ibañez's thirty-five-year-old daughter Cecilia arrived and explained that her mother had been in a state of emotional upset since her father had left home two weeks before. At this Mrs. Ibañez cried out, "No, no! You must not say anything. It's private!" Cecilia quietly replied that she could not stand to see her mother suffer so and that she was frightened by her chest pains. Dr. Mandel then suggested that Mrs. Ibañez might want to talk with the staff psychiatrist. In response she exclaimed, "No! No other people should know about this!" Dr. Mandel drew Mrs. Ibañez closer to him, held her hand, and gently said, "Okay. But we need to talk about this." Cecilia, who was visibly disturbed, pleaded with her mother. "Please, Mama."

Why was Mrs. Ibañez reluctant to discuss the problem that was most likely causing her chest pains? A Mexican nurse on staff later explained that Mexicans feel personal matters should be handled only within the family. They should not be discussed with strangers. Furthermore, a traditional Mexican woman's status is in large part derived from her role as a wife. If her husband leaves, she is nothing. Mrs. Ibañez's pride and embarrassment probably prevented her from talking about the situation. Her daughter, a second-generation Mexican-American, was more Westernized and thus more open with outsiders about personal matters.

As it turned out, Mrs. Ibañez did not have a heart attack and was transferred to the post-coronary-care unit the next day. The nurse attending her case stopped by her room several times before she left. Although she still did not want to discuss her husband, she had stopped crying and was feeling somewhat better emotionally. What she needed most from the staff was nonintrusive warmth and support.

Time Orientation

As discussed in Chapter 1, time orientation refers to an individual's focus on the past, the present, or the future. Most people have a variable time orientation, depending upon the context, but some cultures emphasize one over the others. Countries such as England and China, for example, tend to be past-oriented. That is, they value tradition, doing things the way they have always been done. Individuals from such countries may be reluctant to try new procedures.

People from present-oriented cultures tend to focus on the here and now. They may be relatively unconcerned about the future, expecting to deal with it when it comes. Patients from such cultures—including Latin Americans, Native Americans, and Middle Easterners—may neglect preventive health care measures. They may also show up late, or not at all, for appointments. One such patient was José Velez, a sixty-four-year-old Mexican man.

Mr. Velez made a habit of not showing up for scheduled doctor's appointments and then arriving unexpectedly, requesting that he be seen immediately. He had been diagnosed as having testicular cancer by Dr. Richards three years earlier. Richards had recommended immediate chemotherapy and radiation. Mr. Velez said he would think about it. He missed his follow-up appointment but dropped by Dr. Richards's office several times for pain medication. The doctor, who said he "did not work that way," referred Mr. Velez to home services, with the words, "José needs to understand he has to show up when he is told." Richards refused to see Mr. Velez again and told his nurse to recommend that he take a strong over-the-counter pain reliever.

25

When Sally, the home services nurse, called Mr. Velez to tell him she was coming to see him, he told her not to bother. He did not want to see her unless she brought him pain medication. Sally explained that she had no medication but that perhaps she could help him by telling Dr. Richards he needed something stronger than aspirin. Mr. Velez finally agreed to let her come to his home.

His home was a broken-down toolshed behind some shacks, which he rented for $75 a month. His shower was a garden hose and his bathroom a neighborhood gas station. He slept on a soiled mattress on the floor and kept his clothes in orange crates that doubled as tables and chairs. He had spent the last three years working as a farm laborer and had recently begun collecting recyclable cans and newspapers to support himself.

Sally learned that Mr. Velez had not believed Dr. Richards's diagnosis of cancer three years earlier. He returned to Mexico to seek a *curandero* (native folk healer). Recently, however, a Mexican physician had told him that his only hope for survival was to have his testicles removed. Mr. Velez fled the country. "How can anyone even think that I will allow them to cut my *compañeros* [companions]?" His only family was a distant cousin who lived near his toolshed home in the United States.

Sally spoke with Dr. Richards and explained the situation. Mr. Velez's cancer had advanced. Aspirin could not control the pain. Richards had no sympathy or compassion for Mr. Velez. "He's getting what he deserves. He should have had the surgery when I told him." After several phone conferences, Richards finally agreed to provide a prescription for a stronger pain medication. When Mr. Velez picked it up from the pharmacy, he discovered that the "stronger medication" was merely a ten-day supply of a very mild analgesic.

Richards was punishing his patient for not showing up for his appointments and for not following his advice. He had a total lack of understanding of Mr. Velez's culture. Hispanics tend to have a present time orientation, which is inconsistent with clock time. Getting to an appointment on time takes advance planning. Someone with a strong present time orientation would tend to get involved in the activity of the moment and not think about the time necessary to get somewhere at a particular hour.

Although not necessarily pertinent to Mr. Velez's case, many poor people have difficulty getting time off from work to make an appointment. Public transportation is not always reliable. For the poor, life is often a matter of moment-to-moment survival. Advance planning is a luxury that can often be enjoyed only by those with money.

A final point is that in Latin America, Asia, and other places, most clinics do not make appointments with patients. People come in when necessary and wait to be seen. In addition, Mr. Velez's impatient demand that he see the doctor when he did show up may have been related to his extreme pain.

Mr. Velez's refusal to have his testicles removed was probably related more to his gender's sense of masculinity than to any specific cultural value. Most men seem to identify virility with intact and functioning genitals. I am reminded, however, of a comment I heard about the Mexican notion of machismo. In one of my classes, someone once remarked that machismo was having a big penis. A Mexican student corrected her. "Machismo," she explained, "is having big balls."

Eventually, Mr. Velez was referred to a county facility, where he was treated by a young Hispanic physician who had just spent two years in South America. The two developed a good relationship. Velez was later placed in a hospice, where he died pain-free with his cousin at his bedside and his *compañeros* intact.

Another incident featuring a conflict in time orientation involved Ikem Nwoye, a Nigerian nurse assistant. He would come to the hospital, clock in, and then go to the lounge to have a cigarette and chat. The nurses were often waiting with patients who were signed out and ready to be transferred to Ikem's room. His lack of concern for punctuality created a hardship for the other nurses. They thought he should be fired. They had many difficulties with him, including his inability to take orders from women (which will be discussed in Chapter 5). In such cases, when numerous discussions of the problem fail to resolve it, termination may be the only answer.

I once had an experience with a Native American woman involving present time orientation. I had bought some pottery from her on a trip through the Southwest. A friend admired one of the pots so I decided to try to get her one as a combination Christmas and housewarming present. I had a photograph of the artist holding the pot, which I sent, along with a letter, to the tourist center in her village. I asked if she could make an identical pot for me and, if so, the cost. I gave her my phone number and enclosed a self-addressed stamped envelope.

Two months passed. I assumed that the letter never reached her. Then, late on a Monday afternoon, I got a phone call from her. She was in town for an Indian art show that had been held that weekend. She had made the pot for me and asked if I wanted to pick it up now. She was leaving the city early the next morning.

She was staying on the other side of town, and it was rush hour. I arranged to meet her in the parking lot of a mall later that evening, when the traffic died down. I bought the pot, and my friend loved it. It

26

27

struck me, however, that I had experienced a wonderful, if frustrating, example of present time orientation. The potter might have called or written to let me know she was coming to town. Instead, she waited until the very last moment to call me and make arrangements. She was operating with a present time orientation. She dealt with things when they needed to be done, not before. Many Indian languages, in fact, have no word for time.

Third World cultures often have a present time orientation. Their economies are usually based on agriculture and thus do not require adherence to a clock, an object many people may not even own. It is only in industrialized nations that clock time is important because the performance of everyone's job depends on all others doing theirs. It becomes necessary to adhere to a standard of time.

The weather in such countries is also usually hot. People tend to move more slowly in hot weather than in cold. There is no point trying to rush. People from cold climates, by contrast, tend to be on time. When it is cold, the best way to stay warm is to move quickly. Cold weather countries also tend to be industrialized, and therefore clock time is more important.

Health care professionals can do little about the present time orientation of patients. It is difficult for people who are not used to running their lives by the clock, who think it is rude to interrupt one activity to start another, and whose poverty makes it difficult for them to adhere to other people's schedules to change their ways. The best health care professionals can do is to stress how important it is that patients show up on time for scheduled appointments. But they should be prepared for patients to be late.

When one is dealing with co-workers who operate with a present time orientation, more drastic measures may have to be taken. One person's tardiness can be hard on the rest of the staff and on the patients. If after several discussions and warnings, a tardy staff member does not change, he or she may have to be fired. It is important, however, that everyone realizes that the tardiness is a cultural trait, not a defect in the person's character.

Summary

Miscommunication between health care professionals and their patients often has nothing to do with ethnic background. A common problem is the use of medical jargon, for example, "voided" instead of "peed." Patients may lack the technical vocabulary to describe their symptoms in a way that physicians can understand. Some patients may be very forthright, whereas others may need probing; a health care provider must be sensitive to different communication styles. Patients may be too embarrassed to discuss certain problems, particularly those of a sexual nature. A health care provider needs excellent communication skills to be able to handle sensitive issues.

When the health care provider and the patient are of different ethnic backgrounds, there are numerous additional opportunities for misunderstandings. Communication styles and time orientation vary considerably from culture to culture, causing confusion and sometimes annoyance for hospital personnel. As a further complication, people from different cultures may behave in similar ways but for different reasons. Understanding why people communicate (or do not) in the way they do, however, can help relieve the frustration of health care workers and perhaps contribute to better patient care.

Chapter 3
Religion and Beliefs

It is almost axiomatic that religion is not discussed in polite conversation to avoid the conflicts that stem from different beliefs. Religion is rarely a topic of conversation in hospitals, but religious beliefs and practices are common sources of conflict and misunderstanding. Patients' exercise of their beliefs can result in amusing or even tragic interference with medical care.

Prayer

A seventy-five-year-old Black woman named Agnes Jones was in the hospital recovering from a heart attack. Mrs. Jones was very religious and spent most of her time praying. Her "brothers and sisters" from the church visited daily, and she appeared closer to them than to members of her family.

During her hospital stay, Mrs. Jones consented to only the procedures and medications she believed were ordered by God because according to her world view, only God could make her well. While the nurses bathed Mrs. Jones, she preached to them about Jesus. Before too long, the hospital staff began to avoid her.

For many American Blacks, religion is an essential and integral part of life. God is viewed as the source of both good health and serious illness. He can cure any disease, but to be cured one must pray and have faith. (This world view, like all effective ones, is internally consistent: if a patient is not cured, it is not because God failed but because the patient lacked sufficient faith.)

The hospital personnel did not handle Mrs. Jones's case well. Rather than avoiding her, they should have had a team conference to discuss her beliefs and perhaps invited a minister from her church to attend. The minister might have convinced Mrs. Jones to be more cooperative, and the staff might have learned to be more understanding and tolerant of her beliefs.

29   In another incident, a Filipino nurse named Erlinda went to check on Inez Said, her Iranian patient. When Erlinda entered the room, she found Mrs. Said huddled on the floor, mumbling. At first she thought Mrs. Said had fallen out of bed, but when she tried to help her up, Mrs. Said became visibly upset. Mrs. Said spoke no English, and Erlinda had no idea what the problem was. At that moment, another nurse walked in. Although she was Anglo, she was married to an East Indian Muslim and was able to explain to Erlinda that Mrs. Said had been praying.

Devout Muslims believe they must pray to Mecca, the Holy Land, five times a day. Traditionally, they pray on a prayer rug placed on the floor. Mrs. Said had been kneeling on such a rug. Though most Muslims in the United States use prayer rugs only in the privacy of their homes, devout Muslims in the Middle East take them when they travel. Mrs. Said had come to the United States only a week before and was practicing her religion in the traditional manner. Since she was scheduled for surgery the next day, she thought it was especially important to pray.

Throughout the rest of her hospital stay, Mrs. Said refused to acknowledge Erlinda. She evidently felt that Erlinda might have jeopardized the outcome of her surgery by interrupting her prayers. Fortunately, all went well. If the nursing staff had had some understanding of Muslim customs, they could have arranged to give Mrs. Said privacy during certain times of the day so that she could pray.

30   Another case when religious beliefs and practices caused conflict in a hospital setting involved a group of Gypsies. Their king was in intensive care with dehydration and cardiac arrhythmias. For several days after his admission, the unit was swamped with clan members who chanted loudly and lit candles around the patient's bed. The commotion disrupted the routine of the staff and disturbed other patients. When asked to explain their behavior, the Gypsies said they were trying to keep unwanted spirits from delaying the king's recovery.

Appeals to the king to ask his subjects to be quiet only depressed him. The situation was resolved when he signed himself out of the hospital against medical advice after only four days.

Medical Procedures

31   Religious beliefs can interfere with both the acceptance and the administration of particular medical procedures. Emma Chapman, a sixty-two-year-old Black woman, was admitted to the coronary care unit because she had continued episodes of acute chest pain after two heart

attacks. Her physician recommended an angiogram with a possible cardiac bypass or angioplasty to follow. Mrs. Chapman refused, saying, "If my faith is strong enough and if it is meant to be, God will cure me."

Although Mrs. Chapman never provided any details, she believed she had sinned and her illness was a punishment. According to her beliefs, illnesses from "natural causes" can be treated through nature (e.g., herbal remedies), but diseases caused by "sin" can be cured only through God's intervention. Mrs. Chapman may have felt that to accept medical treatment would be perceived by God as a lack of faith.

Ideally, a staff member would have talked with Mrs. Chapman about her faith, emphasizing that God works through doctors and nurses as well as the patient directly. In this case, medicine could not offer Mrs. Chapman a certain cure; it offered only the possibility of symptom relief and life extension. Someone could have suggested that if she prayed and had enough faith, God would see to it that the operations were successful. She might also have been told the following story:

A huge flood came and destroyed a tiny village. Almost everyone managed to escape in time except for one very religious man who believed that God would save him. He climbed onto his roof to wait. Soon a rescue boat came to help him, but he turned it away, saying, "God will save me." The next day, a second boat came, but again he refused to leave. He said, "My faith in God is strong; He will save me." On the third day, a helicopter flew by to rescue him, and again he turned it away. "God will save me." On the fourth day, the waters rose above his roof and he drowned. When he reached heaven, he demanded to see God. "Why didn't you save me?" he asked. "You've never had a more faithful or loyal servant than I." God responded, "What do you mean? I *did* try to save you. I sent two boats and a helicopter."

Refusing Blood

One of the most common examples of refusing to accept medical help because of a conflict with religious beliefs involves the Jehovah's Witnesses. Most nurses have seen Jehovah's Witness patients refuse blood transfusions for themselves or their children. In some cases, death results. A twenty-three-year-old patient named Barbara Mills developed a pulmonary embolism two weeks after having a baby. She was treated with anticoagulants and was inadvertently over-anticoagulated. This caused her to hemorrhage. She lost so much blood that she needed an immediate blood transfusion. When she refused, the hospital tried to obtain a court order but failed to get one in time. Barbara's

32

hemoglobin level plummeted, and she stopped breathing. She was resuscitated and placed on a respirator.

Until the very end, Barbara refused the transfusion. An elder from the church remained with her, reassuring her that she was in God's hands. When the elder left, her husband panicked and pleaded with the doctors to give her blood. It was too late. Barbara had suffered brain death, stopped assisting the respirator, and died.

33   Sometimes a Jehovah's Witness will reconsider at the last minute. For example, a twenty-seven-year-old woman who began bleeding heavily several days after giving birth required a hysterectomy. After the operation, she urgently needed blood but refused it. Two days later, when she developed acute respiratory distress and had to be placed on a respirator, she agreed to the blood transfusion. It saved her life.

Many health care professionals have strong moral difficulty in respecting the Jehovah's Witness position. The conflict lies in two areas: values and world view. The Jehovah's Witnesses believe that when Armageddon comes, 144,000 of those who have followed God's laws (as interpreted by the Jehovah's Witnesses) will rise from the dead to spend eternity in heaven. Those who have followed His laws but do not go to heaven will spend eternity in a paradise on earth. All those who have violated God's laws (e.g., had a blood transfusion, placed themselves above God by celebrating their own birthdays, or worshiped idols by saluting the American flag) are doomed to spend eternity in nothingness.

Suppose for a moment that they are correct. Choosing to have a blood transfusion can be interpreted as giving up the chance to spend eternity in heaven or paradise in exchange for a few more years on earth. In this scenario, it is not very rational to have a blood transfusion. Few health care professionals are Jehovah's Witnesses. They do not believe that the fate of their soul rests on whether they have a blood transfusion. Thus the world view of Jehovah's Witness patients comes into direct conflict with that of most health care professionals.

Most health care professionals value the life of the physical body. In refusing blood, the Jehovah's Witness is valuing the life of the soul over that of the physical body. The question is, Does any group have the right to impose its values and beliefs on others? Can we be so arrogant and ethnocentric as to be sure we are right and they are wrong?

The issue is most difficult when children are involved. Do their parents have the right to choose for them? This question is not easily answered. In an extreme case, parents abandoned their child after he had been given a blood transfusion under court order.

Finally, there are social issues. If an individual who is a member of a very tightly knit, conservative group of Jehovah's Witnesses accepts blood, the act might lead to rejection by his or her entire social network. A few more years of life may not be worth that price.

Why do some members change their mind and accept blood at the last minute? Obviously, not all members of a religion are equally devout. Many people have doubts about their beliefs. When it is a matter of life and death, faith is often not strong enough to dictate the giving up of life.

Dealing with a Jehovah's Witness patient can be very difficult if the need for a blood transfusion arises. Doctors and nurses often feel helpless and frustrated. They value life so strongly that they find it hard to understand why some people willingly choose to give it up. Perhaps they should try to see the situation from the emic perspective and consider the possibility that the Jehovah's Witnesses are right.

Medical personnel also face conflicts between their duty to patients and their own religious beliefs. In one instance, a nurse of the Jehovah's Witness faith was temporarily transferred to the intensive care unit, where she admitted a patient with gastrointestinal bleeding. He required several units of blood. The nurse refused to hang the blood. It was against her religious beliefs to even participate in a blood transfusion. Reluctantly, she did agree to watch it infuse after someone else started it.

Abortion

Carmen, a Filipino nurse, was informed that she was to be the circulating nurse on a therapeutic abortion. She immediately began to cry and told her supervisor that she would leave work unless her assignment was changed. Carmen was a devout Catholic and refused to participate in an abortion. Joyce, her supervisor, was upset. Other Catholic nurses had worked on abortions before. Besides, she was short of personnel and cases were already running over schedule. Joyce agreed to find someone else to circulate, but she asked Carmen to gather the equipment and supplies for the case. Even this was a problem. "If I set down the room, it's just the same as if I were doing the case," she explained. "I have assisted or aided in taking a life." Joyce finally changed her assignment, but not without some resentment. It is often very difficult for people to understand others' religious practices, especially when they cause inconvenience.

Holy Days

Every religion has days that are considered holy and on which behavior is often strictly proscribed. Sol Meyers, an Orthodox Jew, created a problem for the nursing staff when he tried to observe the Sabbath.

Mr. Meyers brought his wife to the hospital in active labor at 8 P.M. on a Friday. When she gave birth at midnight, the nurses suggested that Mr. Meyers accompany her to the postpartum unit and then return home to rest. He thanked them but explained that he could not drive home because it was the Sabbath. The nurses understood and arranged for him to stay in his wife's room.

In the morning, Mr. Meyers asked the nurses for breakfast. They explained that the hospital provided food only for patients; he would have to buy his breakfast in the dining room. When Mr. Meyers told them he was forbidden to ride in an elevator or handle money, one of the nurses offered to get him food. But Mr. Meyers had no money with him. Frustrated, the nurses finally ordered extra food for his wife to share with him. At lunch, Mr. Meyers once again requested food. This time the nurses suggested that he call a friend or relative to pick him up. Mr. Meyers replied that he could not use the phone on the Sabbath, and even if he made a call, no one would answer because all his friends and relatives were Orthodox. By this time, the nurses were losing patience. If Mr. Meyers could drive to the hospital, why couldn't he drive home? If he knew he would have to stay at the hospital, why had he not brought food with him?

The answers can be found in the Torah. One of the most important laws of the Torah states that Orthodox Jews must observe the Sabbath. It is a time to be with one's family and to worship God. The Sabbath begins at sundown Friday and ends at sundown Saturday. During this time, work of any kind is prohibited, including driving, using the telephone, handling money, and even pushing an elevator button. (A large Jewish hospital in Los Angeles features a few elevators that automatically stop on every floor on Saturday.)

The only law higher than the law of the Sabbath is the law that demands one do everything possible to save a life. Mr. Meyers could drive his wife to the hospital on the Sabbath because her life and that of their child were at stake. He could not drive home, however, because a life was not threatened. Mr. Meyers did not bring food with him because it is forbidden to travel with food on the Sabbath (unless it is milk for a baby). Very little else could have been done in this situation other than to charge extra food to the patient's bill.

37   In another situation involving Jews, a young boy was severely injured one Saturday afternoon while playing football. He needed to go to the hospital immediately. The only person available to take him was his Orthodox grandfather, who drove him the twenty-five miles to the hospital. Once the boy was safely admitted, his grandfather walked home.

Religious Symbols

Religious symbols are not always obvious to members of other reli-   38
gions, and this can lead to problems. In one case, an emergency room
patient named Maria Burlatti needed a chest x-ray. When the technician removed her gown, he found a rosary around Mrs. Burlatti's neck
and asked her to remove it. Mrs. Burlatti was Italian and spoke very
little English. Realizing that she did not understand his request, the
technician attempted to remove the rosary himself, whereupon Mrs.
Burlatti became extremely upset and slapped him. A nursing student
tried to explain to the patient through gestures that her rosary would
be returned as soon as the x-rays were completed, but she still did not
understand. She began to cry.

The head nurse then came upon the scene. She sat beside Mrs.
Burlatti and quietly explained why the rosary had to be removed.
Although she understood the words no better than those of the technician and student nurse, Mrs. Burlatti responded to the calm and sooth-
ing voice. The head nurse gently lifted the rosary off her neck and
placed it on top of Mrs. Burlatti's head. The rosary thus remained in
contact with her body but did not get in the way of the x-rays.

The technician, who was not Catholic, did not realize the rosary
was a religious item and assumed it was a necklace. The patient, who
was ill and scared, needed the symbol of her religious faith more than
ever. Although most Catholics do not wear rosaries, hospital personnel
should realize that older Italian and Mexican women may.

A general rule of thumb is to assume that a patient who is wearing
anything that looks unusual may be doing so for religious reasons.
Hindus may wear sacred threads around their necks or arms; Native
American Indians may carry medicine bundles; Mexican children may
wear a bit of red ribbon; Mediterranean peoples may wear a special
charm on a chain, such as a mustard seed in a blue circle or a ram's
horn, to ward off the evil eye. If an item must be removed to perform a
medical procedure, the reason should be explained to the patient and
the family. The item should be removed gently and respectfully and
kept in contact with the patient's body if possible.

Evil Eye

Belief in the evil eye is widespread throughout Central America, the
Mediterranean, the Middle East, much of Africa, and parts of Asia.
Although the beliefs and associated practices vary, the concept generally includes an evil that one puts on another that causes the victim to
fall ill. The motive is usually envy.

Anthropologists have explained the evil eye curse in terms of the "theory of limited good," which is based on the idea that there is a limited amount of good things in the world, whether beauty, intelligence, wealth, luck, or health. If one person gets more, there is less of it in the world for others. Envy may dictate giving someone the evil eye. The victim's ensuing illness somehow helps even things out.

Belief in the evil eye can create distress and confusion between Mexican and American mothers. In Mexican culture, babies are considered weak and extremely susceptible to the power of an envious glance. It is not even necessary to wish a child harm; a simple compliment, unaccompanied by a touch, can bring on the evil eye. Touching the person while complimenting him or her, however, neutralizes the power of the evil eye.

39   Sue Johnson, a home health nurse, received an angry call from Juanita Garcia, a Mexican-American woman whose house she had visited the day before. As Sue was leaving, she innocently remarked that Mrs. Garcia's child was adorable. The next morning, the infant was crying and feverish. When Mrs. Garcia recalled Sue's compliment and the fact that she had not touched the child, she concluded that Sue had given him the evil eye. Being Anglo, Sue had no knowledge of evil eye. She was innocent, except in the mind of Mrs. Garcia.

Americans are raised to believe that germs cause disease. Mothers are uncomfortable when people get too close to their infants. Mexican mothers, in contrast, may worry when strangers admire their babies without touching them. The very act that is believed to protect a child from illness in one culture is thought to cause illness in another.

Each culture that believes compliments can cause the evil eye also has ways to neutralize them. Putting a bit of saliva on one's finger and making the sign of the cross on a child's forehead when giving a compliment can prevent the evil eye in some (but not all) parts of the Philippines. In Ethiopia, spitting on a child while remarking on its good looks will prevent an inadvertent casting of the evil eye. Not all Mexicans, Filipinos, or Ethiopians adhere to the belief, however, so it is important to pay close attention to nonverbal cues from the mother. Does she appear uncomfortable when you compliment her child? If so, she may believe in the evil eye.

The Color Red

40   A Gypsy king was hospitalized with pneumonia. Members of his clan tied red ribbons to his bed and replaced the standard hospital blanket with a red one. Although this did not create any problem for the hospital staff, it did raise some questions. The Gypsies explained that

the color red is very powerful and can help keep evil spirits away. They were concerned for the health of their king and wanted to do everything they could to help him.

The Garment

Grace Kettering, a Mormon woman, was admitted to the hospital for facial surgery. Before entering the operating room, she was told to remove all her clothes except the hospital gown. She refused to remove her long underwear, and the surgeon refused to operate unless she did.

Devout Mormons who have attained adult religious status in the church wear "the garment." It resembles short-sleeved long underwear and ends just above the knee. Although not exactly magical, it is considered sacred and is always worn except when being cleaned or while one is bathing. Having to remove the garment associated with God's protection can be very distressing to a Mormon patient, especially prior to surgery.

Eventually, Mrs. Kettering's surgeon relented. In such cases, an understanding attitude and a discussion of the options beforehand are advisable. For example, the lower half of the garment could be pulled down to the patient's ankles in the event of abdominal surgery.

Muslim and Arab Dietary Practices

Fatima Bashir, a fifty-year-old Arab Muslim woman, came to the United States for orthopedic surgery. While she was in the hospital, she was served split pea soup as part of her dinner one evening. She became visibly upset and refused to eat the soup. Muslims are forbidden to eat pork. Although the dietary department was told not to serve Mrs. Bashir pork, no one stopped to think that split pea soup contains ham. Careful planning can avoid situations such as this one. Not all such problems, however, are so easily resolved.

An Anglo nurse working in Saudi Arabia encountered a potentially life-threatening dietary problem involving many of her hemodialysis patients. Dates, a favorite food of many Arabs, are very high in potassium, which must be strictly limited in someone suffering from kidney failure. The nurse could not always find an interpreter to explain the situation clearly and convincingly to patients. The situation was further complicated, first, because in Saudi Arabia, food deprivation is considered a precursor to illness. From an Arab's perspective, the nurses were helping to bring on illness by depriving patients of dates. Second, Muslims believe that Allah (God) is all-powerful. Neither dates nor potassium would influence their health; rather, it was God's will. "Inshallah." If Allah meant them to die, so be it. If not, they would survive.

Kosher Dietary Practices

44 Why would a fifty-four-year-old man burst into tears when served meat, milk, and butter on the same lunch tray? What would cause an eighty-seven-year-old woman to refuse beef and chicken, even though she was not a vegetarian? Why would the mother of a two-year-old patient refuse to use the flatware provided and instead insist on plastic utensils? All these individuals are Orthodox Jews following the kosher dietary laws. These laws forbid eating pork and shellfish and nonkosher red meat and poultry, and mixing meat and dairy products, either in the same meal or by using the same plates, pots, or utensils for both.

As with most cultural and religious laws, there is a practical and ideological basis for their origin. The overriding ideology behind the kosher laws is humaneness. The practical reasons are generally associated with health.

Shellfish are to be avoided because they are scavengers. They can pick up diseases and transmit them to the consumer. Pork, if not properly cooked, can cause trichinosis. Furthermore, pigs require shade, water, and human food. In the desert environment it is not a good idea to raise animals that compete with humans for scarce resources. The last two points might explain why Muslims also forbid eating pork. An alternative explanation suggests that because pork and shellfish were dietary staples in the lands where the Jews lived at different points in their history, the taboo was designed to prevent the Jews from integrating. For meat to be considered kosher, animals must be killed with a single blow and not strangled. The pain and suffering an animal experiences between the first and final blows or during the time it takes to die from strangulation can stimulate the release of hormones detrimental to humans. Finally, meat and dairy products should not be combined. Bits of meat may lodge in a wooden or pottery bowl, mix with the dairy products, and in the desert sun provide an ideal breeding ground for bacteria.

Again, the notion of humaneness underlies most of the kosher laws. One can get milk from a living cow or goat, eggs from a living chicken, and wool from a living sheep, but pigs are useful only when dead. To raise an animal strictly for slaughter is considered cruel and inhumane, as is mixing the meat of a calf with the milk of its mother. Finally, the most humane death is one that is instantaneous.

The practical reasons for most of the kosher laws no longer exist. Yet Orthodox Jews continue to uphold the traditions. The behavior of the patients described earlier becomes clear in light of these laws. All these situations can be easily avoided through knowledge of these kosher laws and the use of readily available frozen kosher meal trays and nonreusable paper plates and plastic utensils.

Dietary Practices: Hot and Cold

Nonreligious food restrictions can also create problems. Mina Asami, a sixty-seven-year-old Pakistani woman, was hospitalized with tuberculosis. When Rachel, her nurse, noticed that Mrs. Asami's appetite was poor, she became concerned. Wanting to make sure her patient received enough protein, she made a concerted effort to feed her meat and potatoes with gravy. Mrs. Asami, however, was uncooperative, eating only fruit and jello.

When Mrs. Asami's son Davi came to the hospital, he provided information that resolved the problem. Rachel, it appears, was trying to feed Mrs. Asami foods that Pakistanis normally avoid during the summer. Foods are either hot or cold. These are qualities, not temperatures. In the summer, Pakistanis avoid hot foods like beef because they "make our insides hot." In winter, they avoid cold foods that make their insides cold. Beef, pork, potatoes, and whiskey are all considered hot foods and are avoided in summer; in winter, Pakistanis refrain from eating cold foods such as chicken, fish, fruit, and beer. Once Rachel understood this, she ordered the appropriate foods for Mrs. Asami, who suddenly developed a much heartier appetite.

It is best to ask about food preferences during the admission interview or to arrange for a family member to bring food in for the patient. The latter approach was taken by the family of Chi-Wa Koo, a Chinese patient with lung cancer. A complete Chinese kitchen was laid out on a hospital serving cart. Mr. Koo refused to eat anything prepared by the hospital, consuming only those items brought and prepared by his family.

Mr. Koo's family regarded his lung cancer as a yin or cold condition. To restore balance to his system, it was necessary to give him yang or hot foods. Without a knowledge of yin and yang, it would be impossible for the hospital to serve Mr. Koo the appropriate foods. Furthermore, in China, the family traditionally supplies a patient's food. Fortunately, this incident occurred in a national medical center that is used to treating patients from all over the world. The staff willingly accommodated Mr. Koo's needs by allowing his family to bring in his food.

Food Preferences

Each ethnic group has its own food preferences. Filipinos, for example, like rice with every meal and may feel deprived without it. They sometimes say it is a great comfort to eat rice when they feel ill. Food preferences should be ascertained when a patient is admitted and checked throughout hospitalization because they can have an important psychological effect. Simply discussing the daily menu with the patient can make a significant difference in the patient's attitude and recovery.

Dietary Problems

Some ethnic groups cannot tolerate certain foods. The majority of Asians, Blacks, and Native Americans, for example, are lactose-intolerant, and milk products give them gas and diarrhea. Calcium needs should be considered, however, in planning meals for pregnant women, whether in the hospital or at home. Hispanics generally consider pregnancy a hot condition. Protein-rich foods, which are also usually hot, are avoided during pregnancy to maintain body balance. Physicians should take special care to make sure such women receive adequate protein.

Typical ethnic diets must also be taken into account when discharging patients with special dietary requirements. Asian diets are generally very high in sodium but low in fats. Mexican-Americans tend to use a lot of salt and fats in their cooking. Either of these ethnic cooking styles could prove problematic for hypertensive patients. It may be unrealistic to expect someone to change cooking and eating styles completely. Teaching sessions or adjustment of medications may be necessary. The family cook should be included in all discussions.

Witchcraft

47   Belief in witchcraft is not restricted to remote jungle villages. Carlos Gonzales, a twenty-two-year-old Mexican-American inmate of the county jail, was referred to medical services with symptoms of a heart attack. When the doctor examined him, he discovered no cardiac abnormalities. Carlos was then sent to the mental health section, where he appeared to be in a state of acute fear. He clutched his left side, and his garbled Spanish was incoherent. From his appearance and vital signs, alcohol withdrawal was suspected. He was sent back to the medical service.

Shortly thereafter, Carlos was returned to the mental health service. He lay on the floor, conscious but shaking violently, a look of terror covering his face. He claimed to be dying and begged the nurse to inform his mother. Asking Carlos if he believed in God and getting an affirmative answer, Regina reached for a Bible. She quickly tore out a picture of Jesus and held it over his heart. Slowly he calmed down. When asked if he wanted a cigarette, Carlos surprised everyone by getting up and following Regina to her office.

Still clutching Jesus' picture to his chest, Carlos explained that he had been cursed by a former lover in Mexico. When he ended the relationship, she consulted a *bruja* (witch) who put a spell on him that would cause him to die of a heart attack. Regina called Carlos's home and spoke with his sister, who confirmed the story.

As the night wore on, he gradually stopped shaking but remained fearful. Regina finally convinced Carlos that his belief in God, coupled with the prayers of his family, would counteract the curse. By morning he was fairly calm, perhaps because he was still alive.

Interpreting the incident from an etic perspective, one might suggest that Carlos experienced heartburn that evening. Mindful of the curse, he thought his symptoms signaled a heart attack. His Catholicism may have also contributed to his guilt, punishing his "love" affair with a "heart" attack.

A similar incident occurred in the respiratory intensive care unit. A twenty-four-year-old Mexican-American quadriplegic named Arturo Alvarez was being treated for pneumonia he had developed while in the hospital. Physical therapy was needed to avoid intubation. Arturo, however, was extremely uncooperative. He felt depressed and helpless. In a long conversation with both Arturo and his wife, the head nurse emphasized the importance of physical therapy. She decided to assign Delores, one of her most compassionate nurses and a Mexican-American woman, to Arturo's case.

When Delores first went in to see Arturo, she woke him up to introduce herself and to take his vital signs. When he saw her, he became hysterical and started screaming, *"Bruja, bruja."* He accused Delores of trying to put a spell on him. Apparently he thought she was punishing him for being uncooperative.

Matilda, a psychiatric nurse, was called in. She realized that Arturo really believed he had been hexed. In talking with the family, she learned that his grandmother was thought to have special powers. Matilda obtained the doctor's permission to bring her in to remove the spell.

Arturo's grandmother arrived with several other family members.

48

They surrounded his bed, and the curtain was pulled. Matilda heard moaning in Spanish. Twenty minutes later, the curtain was pulled back, and everyone left except Arturo's wife. Arturo was sleeping peacefully. When he awoke, he was calm, oriented, and cooperative. He agreed to have physical therapy.

Clearly, whatever the grandmother did worked. Whether it functioned as a placebo, as the medical staff believed, or was efficacious in and of itself, as the family believed, is difficult to know. By working within Arturo's belief system, however, the medical staff was able to bring him relief.

Lucky and Unlucky Numbers

Many Americans are superstitious about the number 13. In fact, many buildings lack a thirteenth floor, and many hospitals go from room 12 to room 14 on all wards. Different numbers have positive or negative associations in other cultures.

49

A young Japanese woman named Kieko Ozawa was being wheeled into operating room 4 when she noticed the number over the door. She began to cry softly. The nurse became concerned and asked what was wrong. Kieko was embarrassed but explained that the Japanese character for the number 4 was almost identical to that for the word "death." Already concerned about her health, Kieko was disturbed to be wheeled into a room labeled "death."

Although she said it was just a silly superstition, Kieko was unable to let go of her fear. The surgery went well despite the room number, but the patient suffered needless anxiety. Had the hospital personnel mentioned to Kieko that she was being scheduled for room 4, her feelings might have become known in time to reschedule her into a different operating room. Room number 3, for example, would have been appropriate because 3 in Japanese characters also means "life."

The Chinese regard numbers 8 and 9 as lucky. The character for 8 signifies wealth and the character for 9 means long life. In Hong Kong, most of the expensive luxury cars owned by the Chinese include the number 8 on the license plate. The Chinese pay extra money and wait in long lines to get a plate with that number. An expensive car without an 8 is generally owned by a foreigner.

Whereas the number 4 has negative connotations for the Japanese, the opposite is the case for the Navaho, who see much of the world in terms of four. Phrases are repeated four times in their ritual chants, pollen is thrown to the four directions in many of their ceremonies, and they revere four sacred mountains. A Navaho might find it easier to remember to take medicine four times a day than three or five times.

Obviously, health care workers cannot be expected to know all the superstitions of every ethnic group. What is important to remember is that superstitions are a part of every culture and may surface during the emotionally trying times of illness. Problems can be avoided by giving patients as much information as possible in advance and then by being sensitive to their reactions.

Astrology

Numbers are significant for believers in astrology. Ngoc Ly, a twenty-five-year-old Vietnamese man, was hit by a car while riding his bicycle to work. Paramedics were able to resuscitate him, but the physician at the local trauma center determined that Ngoc was clinically brain dead. He placed him on life support until Ngoc's family could be notified.

An interpreter explained Ngoc's condition to his wife and parents. They nodded in understanding and quietly left the hospital. Normally, the staff neurosurgeon would then have pronounced Ngoc dead and removed him from the ventilator, but he was suddenly called to surgery.

Later that afternoon, Ngoc's family met with Dr. Isaacs, the physician they had spoken to earlier. Isaacs intended to tell them of the plan to pronounce Ngoc dead and discontinue the ventilator, but the Lys had other plans. They informed him that they had consulted a specialist who said this was not the right time for Ngoc to die. Dr. Isaacs was confused. What specialist would make such a recommendation? An astrologer who had read Ngoc's lunar chart advised that his death be postponed until a more auspicious date.

The physician had never encountered a situation like the one now facing him. Fearing legal repercussions if he did not abide by the family's request, he agreed to keep Ngoc on life support until further notice. A little less than a week later, the Lys called to tell him that Ngoc could now die.

Most members of the staff were stunned by this incident. Ngoc's body was starting to decompose and smell. People looked up books on astrology and questioned Vietnamese co-workers. They learned that astrology is taken seriously by many Asians. When an important decision is to be made, they will often consult a *bomoh* or *dukun* to interpret the astrological charts.

Although most people cannot predict or control the date of their death, simply knowing when someone has died can be helpful in terms

50

of knowing what fate has in store for the deceased's descendants. If a person dies at the "proper" time, his or her children will be rewarded with good health and goodwill. If the time is inauspicious, the children will suffer financial losses, unhappy marriages, or similar negative fates. A *bomoh* can tell people what the future holds for them so they can be prepared.

The Ly family had an opportunity denied to most people. By delaying removal of Ngoc's life support, they could influence the fate of his descendants for generations. How could they not do everything possible to bring good luck to his children?

Death and Candles

51   Philip Maturo, a Gypsy king in his late seventies, was brought to the hospital and diagnosed with pneumonia. The severity of his illness necessitated an oxygen tent. Clan members caused pandemonium; they crowded into Mr. Maturo's room, blocked the doorways, and filled the cafeteria with their coffee cups and cigarette smoke. This behavior, however, was merely a nuisance. The greatest problem was that they insisted on keeping a candle on the shelf at the head of Mr. Maturo's bed. The nurses lived in fear that it would be lit while the oxygen was turned on and cause an explosion. Many animated discussions were held on this point, but the Gypsies were adamant. If their king died, the candle would be lit at the moment of death to guide his spirit to heaven. Fortunately, Mr. Maturo recovered and the hospital survived.

52   Another hospital witnessed a different Gypsy custom regarding death. When the end was imminent, the clan received the hospital's permission to move the king outside, bed and all. They felt this would help free the soul of their dying leader, now unencumbered by walls and ceilings.

A Dying Queen

53   The staff at another hospital faced a different problem when a dying Gypsy queen was a patient in its intensive care unit. Several Gypsy women kept a vigil at Sylvia Romany's bedside, blocking the nurses' access. Finally, one of them explained that when the queen dies, her powerful soul will enter the body of the person physically closest to her. The women were all vying for that position. They certainly would not want her soul to enter the body of one of the nurses. The staff was frustrated, but there was little they could do for Mrs. Romany in any case. She died a few days later, and presumably her soul entered the body of the most determined Gypsy woman.

Summary

Although conflicting belief systems can be a source of frustration, confusion, and misunderstanding, most can be dealt with successfully. One must understand the patient's beliefs and be willing to respect them. When health care personnel work *with* the patient's beliefs, rather than against them, the outcomes are usually more successful, measured not only in patient satisfaction but also in ease for the medical team in managing the patient and family.

Chapter 4
Family

A nurse when asked what is the most common problem she encounters when dealing with non-Anglo ethnic groups will likely answer, "Their families."

Visitors

A sixty-five-year-old Filipino woman named Carlita Ricos lay dying for six months. Although she was in a coma, her fourteen children were with her constantly, bathing her, grooming her, rubbing her favorite lotion on her skin. Her failure to respond did nothing to diminish their devotion. The nursing staff reacted in several ways. Many were impressed with the dedication of the Ricos family. Others were annoyed by the constant stream of visitors. Few understood why Mrs. Ricos's family spent so much time with her.

Filipinos have great respect for their parents. They feel they owe an eternal debt of prime obligation—*utang na loob*—to their parents for giving them life and making sacrifices for them. Mrs. Ricos's children felt they owed their mother all the time and care they could give. They never considered that they might be in the nurses' way.

A similar incident involved a Chinese family. Very early one morning, before the sun had arisen, Chi-Fan Wong's nurse, Nancy, stumbled over a body curled up on the floor. When her eyes grew accustomed to the darkness, she discovered two other people sleeping on a cot and in the chair. Mr. Wong's wife was standing at his bedside, holding her husband's glass while he swallowed his medications. Nancy soon discovered a serving cart, covered with food prepared by his family. Later that afternoon, another group of family members arrived, and the original group went home to rest.

Until the night Mr. Wong died, someone was with him at all times. The visitor's chair served as a bed. His wife and sons bathed him, fed him, and massaged his body. Interestingly, his sons were more involved in his care than his daughters. In an almost identical situation, Sam Inouye, a Japanese patient in his late fifties, was constantly attended by his wife and children. They took over all his personal care, a service usually provided by the nurses.

The custom in both China and Japan is for the family to take care of the patient's personal needs. The medical staff is there to practice medicine. Both respect and obligation require that children minister to their parents.

The Asian respect for parents can be illustrated by the following hypothetical situation. You are in a boat with your mother and your child when the boat capsizes. You can save only one person. Whom do you save? Most Americans would respond, "My child," reasoning that their mother had lived her life whereas their child's was just beginning. Most Asians perceive the situation differently. They would more likely respond, "My mother," explaining that they can always have another child, but they can have only one mother.

The different perspectives also reflect a difference in family relationships. Traditionally, most Asians live in extended family households and tend to value the family of orientation (the individual, parents, and siblings) above the family of procreation (the individual, spouse, and children). Sons generally live with their parents until they die, and that long-term relationship takes precedence over any other. In contrast, Americans usually live in nuclear family households. Ties to parents are weakened after marriage, while those to spouse and children are strengthened. The choice of whether to save the mother or child reflects the traditionally stronger familial tie.

The reason Mr. Wong's sons were more involved in his care than his daughters is that Chinese were traditionally patrilocal; that is, sons continued to live with their parents after marriage. It was their obligation to care for their aging progenitors. Daughters, however, moved in with their in-laws. Their primary responsibility was to their husbands' parents, not their own. Therefore, in an extension of traditional residence patterns, we find the man's sons at his bedside, rather than his daughters.

A Laotian family rarely left the room of their six-year-old son. He was in intensive care after falling under a moving car. Although visitors are to be kept at an absolute minimum in this unit, at least two family members were there all the time. The nurses' job was made even more difficult because the room was small and filled with a great deal of equipment. The nurses also complained that they felt they were being watched by the family, which made them feel uncomfortable.

Like other Asian groups, Laotians have very strong family support systems. It is important for them to take care of each other when ill. This family had come to the United States only two years previously, after suffering many traumatic separations during the war in Southeast Asia, and may not have been ready to trust authority figures by leaving the child alone in the staff's care.

Asians are not the only ethnic group that hovers around the sickbeds of their relatives. The entire family of a sixteen-year-old Mexican-American youth crowded in the hospital waiting room while he was being treated for minor injuries. A friend had brought him into the emergency room at 1:30 A.M. He had been injured in a gang fight. Fortunately, the contusions and lacerations he received were not serious; few stitches were required. Nevertheless, well over a dozen relatives—including aunts, uncles, and cousins—arrived at the hospital and remained by his side until he was released.

Gypsies cause some of the worst complaints regarding family visitors. For example, when Louis Romano, king of his clan, became ill, thirty to fifty of his relatives, friends, and "elders" literally took over the small hospital where he was a patient in intensive care. They came in the evening and stayed all night, despite the posted notice that visiting hours were limited. The Gypsies who were not in the patient's room or lobby roamed the parking lot. Everyone in the hospital—supervisors, security, maintenance, office staff, and nurses—tried in vain to maintain order, politely explaining procedure and protocol, but without effect.

Gypsies live within a large extended family unit known as a clan. All members are considered immediate family. When any member is ill, it is important to show respect and concern through one's presence. Because the patient in this case was the king, the attendance of the entire clan was almost mandatory. A few elders even came from across the country to be with him.

Gypsies are commonly nomadic, traveling in groups. When they enter a hospital, that becomes their temporary home. If possible, Gypsy patients should be put in private rooms at the end of a hall so as to minimize traffic problems and disturbance to other patients. Other than that, hospital staff must be prepared for a constant stream of people moving into the hospital to be near the patient.

One reason large numbers of ethnic family members who visit patients and often remain twenty-four hours a day create significant difficulties for hospital staff is that American hospitals were built by

Americans for Americans. Americans tend to have small families and to live in nuclear family households. Furthermore, privacy is a major American value. Generally few family members live near enough to the hospital to come visit very often. When they do, they usually stay for only a short period of time because they feel the patient should be left alone to rest in order to get well. Therefore, hospital rooms rarely have more than one visitor's chair per bed and visiting hours may be extremely limited. Second, Americans value money as well as privacy. Hospitals are a business. If there is room for another bed, it should be for a patient, not for a family member who wants to sleep over.

Hospitals in other cultures are designed and run differently. Patients are expected to have several visitors. A cot is usually provided for anyone who spends the night. Privacy is not a concern.

60   Betsy Sanders, a former student, broke her leg in a skiing accident in Spain. The doctor at the clinic told Betsy that her ligaments were shredded but that he could correct the condition with surgery. When Betsy awoke from surgery, she was nauseated and in terrible pain but could not vomit. She was too embarrassed. There were ten people in the room waiting to see her. She was in a large private room, and a couch had been turned into a guest bed. All her friends in Spain had gotten together and decided Betsy should never be left alone. They worked out a visiting schedule. One friend even took a leave of absence from work to be with her.

Although Betsy appreciated their concern, their solicitousness made her uncomfortable. All but one of her friends were male. She was in bed with her leg in the air for two weeks, wearing nothing but a little gown. She had to be washed in bed and use a bedpan. She could not wash her hair or even brush her teeth. She looked awful and felt worse. All she wanted was to be left alone.

Her situation was the reverse of the non-Anglo in an American hospital. The hospital staff expected her to have visitors around the clock and provided a bed for that purpose. Her friends assumed she would want company and ignored what they interpreted as her polite protestations that she would be fine if left alone. She did not have any family in Spain so they were filling in. They would have wanted the same attention had the situation been reversed. In this case, however, what the patient longed for was some privacy.

In summary, then, hospitals are designed with the needs and values of the culture in mind. Problems arise when the patient is of a different ethnic group, with a different set of values and needs. In a country like the United States, with its huge population of non-Anglo residents, this is frequently the case. It is important to remember that the patient is not just an individual but a member of a family. When one member is ill, the entire group is affected. Ideally, the family can help care for the patient, freeing the staff for more technical medical care.

A related problem that frequently arises is the failure of many non-Anglo patients to care for themselves.

Self-Care

Tome Tanaka, a Japanese man in his sixties, was a patient in the rehabilitation unit. A stroke had left him with significant weakness on his left side. Self-care was an important part of his therapy. He had to relearn to feed himself, dress, shave, use the bathroom, and do other daily activities. Kathy, his nurse, spent a great deal of time carefully explaining to Mr. Tanaka how the staff would work with him on these tasks. The patient and his wife listened passively; his children and grandchildren appeared more interested. Several hours later, when Mr. Tanaka's children and grandchildren left, Kathy came into the room and discovered Mrs. Tanaka waiting on her husband as though he were an invalid.

She was not alone in impeding his progress, however. He refused to do anything for himself and continually barked commands at her. Rather than use the toilet, he insisted that she hold the bedpan for him. He refused to brush his teeth, shave, or dress, demanding that his wife do everything for him.

Mr. Tanaka attended physical therapy and occupational therapy sessions each day and did quite well. He learned to walk with a cane. He needed minimal assistance with self-care activities. Despite his progress in therapy, however, as soon as his wife or one of his children arrived, he regressed. He was discharged after four weeks, almost as dependent as when he first came.

Kathy and the other nurses were frustrated over Mr. Tanaka's dependency, especially when they saw that he was capable of taking care of himself. They took his "failure" personally, as though they were not doing their jobs properly. What might the nurses have done differently? First, they needed to understand that patients and their families do not always share the same goals as health care personnel. Second, they might have allowed the family to observe Mr. Tanaka during physical and occupational therapy sessions. Unlike most hospitals, this one barred families from such sessions because of the potential distraction for the patient. In this case, the rule might have been waived.

Juan Martinez, a thirty-six-year-old Mexican man with second-degree burns on his hands and arms, posed a similar problem. The skin grafts had healed, and there was now danger that the area would

61

62

stiffen and the tissue shorten. The only way to maintain maximum mobility was through regular stretching and exercise. The nurses explained to Mr. Martinez's wife that feeding himself was an essential therapeutic exercise. The act of grasping the utensils and lifting the food to the mouth stretches the necessary areas. Mrs. Martinez seemed to understand the nurses' explanation, yet she continued to cut her husband's food and put it in his mouth.

When Linda, one of his nurses, observed this, she took the fork out of Mrs. Martinez's hand and told Mr. Martinez to feed himself because he needed to exercise his arms and hands. Linda again explained to Mr. Martinez's wife how important it was for him to do it himself. Mrs. Martinez appeared skeptical but did not argue. Mr. Martinez looked at Linda peevishly and made a feeble attempt at eating. His wife watched with pity. Linda knew from seeing Mr. Martinez when his wife was not around that he was perfectly capable of feeding himself. Linda left the room. When she looked in five minutes later, she saw Mrs. Martinez once again cutting her husband's food and putting it in his mouth.

63   Jong Kim, a forty-seven-year-old Korean man, was hospitalized with fractured lower legs and pelvis. He demanded that the nurses feed and bathe him. He was physically able to do some of these tasks; he simply did not want to. When the nurses refused, he waited for his wife or daughters to do so. The nurses set up his meals, expecting him to feed himself. He let the food get cold until his wife arrived and could feed it to him. Mrs. Kim also brought in special foods for her husband to eat.

The nurses were irritated by Mr. Kim's demands for assistance with tasks he could do himself. Fortunately, a Korean nurse on staff was able to explain to the other nurses that Korean men expect to be waited on. Having Mr. Kim's family available to care for him most of the time also eased their burden.

Failure to care for oneself is common in cultures that emphasize the family over the individual—in other words, almost all cultures other than Anglo-American. Self-care is important to Americans in part because we value independence so highly. In contrast, Asian and Hispanic cultures emphasize family interdependence over independence. For them, self-care is not an important concept.

In many cases, Americans' ethnocentrism blinds them to the fact that life in a typical Asian or Hispanic household may be different from that in the normal Anglo home. Self-care may be a practical necessity in the Anglo home, where there may be no one to help the former patient with such tasks. In contrast, many Asians and Hispanics live in large extended family households, where someone is usually at home to care for the patient.

Another significant factor is the difference between egalitarian and hierarchical cultures. In an egalitarian culture such as our own, everyone is theoretically equal. And, theoretically, no one in the family is considered subservient to anyone else. In hierarchical Asian cultures, some members of the family are clearly dominant (males and elders) while others are clearly subordinate (females and children). The case studies involving the Tanakas and Kims illustrate the proper roles of wife and children in hierarchical cultures. It is their duty to obey and care for the dominant family member—the husband and father.

In the situation with the Martinez couple, duty plays a less prominent role. It is of greater importance that when a family member is ill, love and concern are demonstrated through care and attention. The nurses might have instructed Mrs. Martinez to help her husband in ways that would not hinder his rehabilitation. For example, they could have showed her how to massage lotion onto his hands.

Control may also play a role in the failure to care for oneself. Each of the situations described above involved a man whose culture clearly acknowledged his power and authority. All of these men, however, were reduced to a state of physical weakness by their medical condition. Ordering people around and having them wait upon one's every need are ways of demonstrating dominance. It may masquerade as helplessness, but it is a way of maintaining control.

The hospital staff often has conflicts with family members over issues other than self-care or too many visitors.

Perceived Discrimination

The patient was a ten-month-old Black male. His hands and feet were tied to the bed to prevent him from pulling out the intravenous lines. When Mrs. Wilson, his grandmother, saw him tied down, she became very angry. "How come you got the baby tied down? He's not doing anything. He ain't no trouble. Why don't you untie him? He looks like he can't move. He ain't no dog!" She had experienced much discrimination at the hands of whites and perceived her grandson's treatment as a racist act. Once the nurse explained the purpose of tying the baby down, she relaxed.

64

Gifts

A more pleasant problem arose during a Korean woman's discharge. Mrs. Chow had been cared for during her week in the hospital by a nurse named Florine. Florine frequently stopped in to see Mrs. Chow, offering to help in any way she could to make her patient more com-

65

fortable. Mrs. Chow's family was often there and observed Florine's kindness. When Mrs. Chow was being discharged, her twenty-five-year-old son, Jim, took Florine aside and gave her some money. Florine thanked him but refused it, explaining that she could not accept money for doing her job. Furthermore, it was against hospital policy. He insisted that she take it and put it in her pocket. "My mother wants you to have this. She wants to thank you." Florine took the money from her pocket, this time more adamant in her refusal. Jim in turn became extremely embarrassed.

In Korea, it is common for the family to give a patient's nurse food, money, or a special gift to show gratitude for the care she is giving. For Florine to refuse the gift was both insulting and improper. Reciprocity is important in many Asian cultures. When someone does something for another, something is owed in exchange. If the exchange is not completed, the person receiving the kindness is in the other's debt. Since this is an uncomfortable position to be in, it is extremely important not to let such indebtedness occur. A gift to the nurses satisfies the reciprocal obligation.

The stalemate ended when Florine told Jim to take the money and buy some candy for all the nurses to share. This suggestion took care of the Chow family's need to show their appreciation and allowed Florine to adhere to her own values and hospital policy.

The families of Jewish patients also often give nurses gifts while the patient is in the hospital. It is not done so much through a feeling of obligation and reciprocity, however, than as a way of ensuring good care.

Whatever the reason, when a family member presents a gift to the nurse, she will create a great deal of awkwardness if she refuses it. The solution most commonly practiced is for the nurse to share the gift with all the other nurses on the floor.

Informed Consent and Kinship

A final family problem involves the issue of who should sign informed consents. Legally, only the parents or legal guardian of a child may sign. In some cultures, however, other persons might be more appropriate—a Navaho boy's grandparent or maternal uncle, for example.

It is not uncommon for Native American grandparents to raise their grandchildren while the parents leave the reservation to work. As the child's primary caretaker, a grandparent might bring a child in to the hospital. Legally, however, the grandparent would not be able to sign a consent form for the child.

The role of the Navaho maternal uncle is a bit more complicated.

It is based on the kinship structure of Navaho society. American kinship structure is *bilateral;* we are equally related to members of both sides of our family. Social ties might be closer to one side, but the legal relationship is identical. Many other cultures are *unilineal,* that is, they trace their descent from either a male or a female ancestor. A member of a patrilineal culture (such as many in the Middle East) is considered a member of the father's family, rather than the mother's. In contrast, a member of a matrilineal culture (such as the Navaho or Hopi) is a member of the mother's family, rather than the father's.

Although women tend to have greater power and respect in matrilineal societies than in patrilineal ones, property is passed on from male to male. In matrilineal societies, a boy will inherit from his closest male relative. In this case, it will be his *mother's brother,* because the boy is not considered a member of his father's family. His father will pass on any property or privileges to his own sister's children. Genetically, this arrangement makes sense. A boy always shares the genes of his mother's brother. It is not so certain that he will carry those of his mother's husband. It is not hard to imagine a situation in which a Navaho man might bring his nephew into the hospital, only to be told he is not empowered to sign an informed consent.

Summary

Family structure and relationships are not the same in every culture. In many cases, accommodation will be difficult, if not impossible, given hospital architecture, American medical values, and the American legal system. At the very least, however, greater understanding of the ways of other cultures may have a positive effect on the attitudes of those providing patient care.

Chapter 5

Men and Women

Sex and gender are frequent sources of conflict and misunderstanding. Not every culture has been affected by the women's movement. Few share the American ideal of equality between the sexes.

Informed Consent

A twenty-six-year-old Mexican woman named Rosa Gutierrez brought her two-month-old son to the emergency room. Rosa was concerned because he had diarrhea and had not been nursing. The staff discovered that he was also suffering from sepsis, dehydration, and high fever. The physician wanted to perform a routine spinal tap, but Rosa refused to allow it. When asked why, she said she needed her husband's permission before anything could be done to the baby. The staff tried to convince her that this was a routine procedure, but Rosa was adamant. Nothing could be done until her husband arrived.

Although legally Rosa could have signed the consent, culturally she lacked the authority. In the traditional Mexican household, the man is the head of the family and makes all major decisions. Rosa was unwilling to violate that norm. Fortunately, her husband soon arrived and signed the informed consent.

Women and Authority

An Iranian mother and father admitted their thirteen-month-old child, Ali, to the pediatrics unit. After three days of rigorous testing and examination, it was discovered that Ali had Wilms tumor, a type of childhood cancer. Fortunately, the survival rate is 70 to 80 percent with proper treatment.

66

67

Before meeting with the pediatric oncologist to discuss Ali's treatment, Mr. and Mrs. Mohar were concerned and frightened, yet cooperative. Afterward, however, they became completely uncooperative. They refused permission for even the most routine procedures. Mr. Mohar would not even talk with the physician or the nurses. Instead, he called other specialists to discuss Ali's case.

After several frustrating days, the oncologist decided to turn the case over to a colleague. He met with the Mohars and found them extremely cooperative. What caused their sudden reversal in behavior? The fact that the original oncologist was a woman.

Even though the Mohars had described themselves as "Americanized," the Iranian tradition of male authority was still strong. They could not accept a woman making life-and-death decisions for their son. Ali's treatment was too important to be decided by a woman.

Several weeks later, it became necessary to insert a permanent line into Ali to administer his medication. The nurse attempted to show Mrs. Mohar how to care for the intravenous line, but Mr. Mohar stopped her. "It is *my* responsibility only. You should never expect my wife to care for it." Throughout each encounter with the hospital staff, Mrs. Mohar remained silent. She deferred to her husband.

Interestingly enough, the nurses had few problems with the Mohars. They were treated with respect because, as Mr. Mohar stated, they were functioning under the direction of the physician. Their only problem was in understanding why the Mohars initially refused treatment for Ali. They had assumed that since both parents were educated in American universities and had described themselves as Americanized, they really were. The stress of their son's illness, however, had made them revert to traditional ways. The importance of male dominance in the Middle East is also a major factor in the following situations.

Male Dominance

68   Nader and Shahab, two healthy looking Iranian men in their late twenties, came into the emergency room demanding to see a doctor. Julie, the nurse on duty, asked what the problem was. Nader curtly responded that he wanted to see a doctor, not a nurse. Julie calmly explained that he first had to be assessed by a nurse. Nader and his friend did not want to wait, however. Julie said they became loud, pushy, and insulting. Roberta, another nurse, came on the scene and told them that Nader did not appear to be seriously ill and would have to be patient. The doctor would see him soon. Nader then stormed past

the two nurses, headed into the patient area, and demanded to see a doctor immediately. The nurses had to call security.

What caused Nader's behavior? He felt he warranted the attention of a male doctor, not a mere female nurse. He also probably felt uncomfortable talking with a woman about his problem. He had a venereal disease.

Later, Nader telephoned the emergency room and asked for Julie. "My friend and I have quite a bit of money. Why don't you and another nurse join us?" Needless to say, Julie did not accept his proposition. She was mystified as to what gave him the impression that she would even consider going out with him. Julie had probably made eye contact with Nader, creating the impression that she was sexually "loose" and interested in dating him.

Aggressiveness

Nurses often comment on the aggressiveness of Middle Easterners, whether they be Arab, Iranian, or Israeli. Cultural norms of behavior are generally dictated by circumstances. Life in the Middle East is extremely difficult, both environmentally and politically. Survival in this harsh climate requires toughness, aggressiveness, even pushiness. Such behavior works there. The environment in the United States is different. Assertiveness is admired while aggressiveness is not. But it is usually hard to change a personal style that has been effective in the past.

Domineering Husbands

A nineteen-year-old Saudi Arabian woman named Sheida Nazih had just given birth. Her husband, Abdul, had been away on business during most of their ten-month marriage but brought her to the United States to have their baby. He moved into the hospital room with Sheida immediately after she gave birth. He kept the door to their room shut and questioned everyone who entered, including the nurses. The nurses were not happy with this procedure but felt they had no choice except to comply.

Although Sheida could speak some English, the only time she would speak directly to the nurses was when Abdul was out of the room. Otherwise, he answered all questions addressed to her. He also decided when she would eat and bathe. As leader of the family, Abdul felt it was his role to act as intermediary between his wife and the world.

69

Domineering Sons

70   The mother of a three-year-old Egyptian boy named Mohammad was completely unable, or unwilling, to discipline him. He was hospitalized following surgery for a closed reduction of a leg fracture sustained in an accident. Rather than bring the boy to the recovery room after surgery, it was decided to let him recover in a crib in his hospital room. The staff thought he would do better there because he was so young. His parents could be with him when he awoke.

Diane, the nurse, had a surprise waiting for her when she brought Mohammad to his room. Not only were his parents there, but aunts, uncles, cousins, neighbors, and even one of his small friends. An Egyptian neighbor, fluent in English, explained that in Egypt, when anyone was sick enough to be in the hospital, the entire family came to provide moral support. When Diane asked him to tell everyone to wait in the lobby, he complied.

Leili, Mohammad's mother, sat by her son's crib. As he began to wake from the anesthesia, she spoke softly to him. As he awakened more fully, however, he became unruly. Leili could not handle him, and his father made no effort. The father had been charged with watching Mohammad when the accident occurred so he may have felt some guilt, which affected his behavior.

Diane had hoped that when Mohammad's intravenous catheter was removed he would calm down. She did not expect a small boy to be well behaved under such circumstances. Unfortunately, removing the intravenous line allowed him to use his now freed hand to try to hit his mother and Diane. Throughout Mohammad's recovery period, he appeared to dominate Leili. She made no effort to correct his behavior. Although it is difficult to guess at the interpersonal dynamics involved, Leili may have been lenient with the boy in part because of his status as a first-born male in a male-dominated culture.

Elders in Charge

71   The parents of an eight-year-old Gypsy boy named Tony Romano also lacked authority over their son, but in a different way. He was afflicted with Guillain-Barré syndrome and had lost control over all his muscles, including those of his respiratory system. Whenever the male physician asked to speak with the parents, the paternal grandmother and two aunts insisted that he speak with them instead. The grandmother said she did not want the parents to see the child. When the issue of signing informed consent forms came up, the grandmother said they would have to wait until her husband arrived.

Shortly thereafter, a meeting was called with the physician, the two grandfathers, a great-grandfather; and a few uncles. The parents were excluded from the conference by the elder males, who later had the father sign the consent form. The grandmothers were excluded without discussion. It was assumed that only the elder males would take part.

Family members did not allow the Romanos to see their child until two days after his admission, when his condition had stabilized. When his mother finally saw Tony, she became hysterical. The group forbade her to see him again for a while. Family members frequently asked the staff for information about the child's condition, but all decisions were made by Tony's grandfather.

One of the nurses finally asked Tony's grandmother why the boy's parents were not allowed to see him or talk with the physicians. She explained, "They are too young. They are just babies." Tony's father was twenty-eight, his mother twenty-four.

Gypsy marriages are often arranged when the couple are in their mid-teens. After marriage, they usually live with the husband's parents and are sheltered from adult responsibilities and decisions for many years. Wisdom is thought to come with age. The Romanos were still considered children despite the fact that they were parents.

This attitude was very difficult for the nurses to accept. Anglo-American culture expects parents to assume full responsibility for their children, no matter what their age. Legal consent for medical procedures may be given only by the parents. Information regarding a child's condition is given only to the parents. In some cases, only the parents are allowed to visit the child. It was very disconcerting for the nurses to have all the rules changed, but the Gypsies insisted on doing things their own way.

The fact that all the important decisions were made by the men, with no input from the women, is also cultural. Gypsies have a male-dominated (and age-dominated) society. Women are not allowed to interrupt men's conversations, let alone join them in making decisions.

Authority Figures

Knowing who holds the position of authority can help resolve difficult situations. The following incident also involved a group of Gypsies. It began late one night when Maria, aged about eighteen, came into the hospital to deliver her baby. The infant was very small and required special care. The next morning, Rosalyn, Maria's nurse, got a call from the nursery. Three women had just shown up, all claiming to be the baby's mother. None of them was a patient, and all were well over the age of eighteen.

Rosalyn immediately went to the nursery, where the other nurse pointed her out to the three women and fled. The youngest woman said, "That's our baby. We want him." The next one agreed. The oldest woman, Helena Tabiri, looked at Rosalyn and asked if she was the boss. Rosalyn answered affirmatively and asked how she could help her. Mrs. Tabiri said, "The baby is the son of my daughter. My family is responsible for this child. I will take him home and care for him."

Rosalyn explained that Maria would be taught to care for him. Mrs. Tabiri asked that the lessons begin immediately. Her request was denied. The baby needed to remain in the hospital for a few more days. She then asked to see the baby. Rosalyn showed him to her and thought that was the end of the incident.

She was wrong. A few hours later, Rosalyn got another call from the postpartum floor. The three women had gone to Maria's room, where a loud argument had ensued. The next time the nurse checked her room, Maria was gone, along with everything movable. While she was on the postpartum floor, Rosalyn got a call from the nursery. The three "mothers" were back, along with at least twenty-five other people. They were all crowded around the window outside the nursery. When Rosalyn informed Mrs. Tabiri that Maria was missing, she replied, "She is not missing. She is home where she belongs." Mrs. Tabiri added that she had come to take the baby home. Rosalyn quickly called over one of the pediatricians to explain to Mrs. Tabiri why the baby needed to stay in the hospital. His explanation was convincing, and Mrs. Tabiri agreed.

The relatives of the newborn Gypsy crowded around the window of the nursery. Although individuals came and went, there were always about twenty people there, making it difficult for people who wanted to see other babies. When Rosalyn politely asked them to leave room for other families, they ignored her.

The situation was resolved when the Gypsy king arrived. Rosalyn explained the situation to him. "Are you telling us to leave?" he asked, giving her a menacing look. She assured him that she only wanted to let others through. He smiled and said he would talk to his people.

From that point on, they were no trouble. He was the leader, and his directives were considered binding, unlike those of the nurse, who was both a woman and an outsider. When the physician said the baby could be discharged, Rosalyn went to the king and told him the baby's natural mother would have to come in for the child. He said he would handle it. Maria arrived later that evening to take her baby home.

Had Rosalyn appealed to the group as a whole, it is unlikely that they would have complied. She recognized, however, that the king was the authority figure, and by gaining his cooperation, she was able to maintain some control. The two aberrant aspects of the situation involved Mrs. Tabiri and her daughter Maria. Mrs. Tabiri was a strong woman in a male-dominated culture. In the absence of men, she appeared to be making decisions. Furthermore, it was unusual for Maria to have arrived alone for her delivery. She may have been out and gone into labor unexpectedly. The absence of a husband and the strong role played by her mother (as opposed to her mother-in-law) may indicate that Maria was not married; it is unclear. In any case, these two deviations should serve as an important reminder that people are individuals, not simply representatives of their culture, and may act in ways contrary to cultural norms.

In many cultures, including Gypsy, Asian, Middle Eastern, and Hispanic, males are authority figures. Unless they are very Westernized, it is often best to consider them as the spokespersons for the family. They are generally the ones who will make the decisions. This recommendation may be difficult for those with feminist leanings, but it is likely to be the most productive approach. Age is also a sign of authority in Gypsy and Asian cultures so initial conversations should be addressed to the eldest male.

It is unwise, however, to assume that males are always in charge. In matrilineal cultures such as the Navaho, the oldest women may have the greatest authority and decision-making power. The same may be true in many Black families. Although Black Americans are not matrilineal, the structure of the single-parent family household may lead to the same result.

Dominant and Subordinate Roles

Traditional dominant and subordinate roles can also create friction 73 among hospital staff. For example, Ikem Nwoye, the Nigerian male nurse assistant discussed in Chapter 2, would have what one nurse described as a temper tantrum whenever a female registered nurse asked him to do something. Other times he would sulk and simply leave the room. What he would not do is take instructions from a woman. In Nigeria, men are considered superior to women. Men tell women what to do, not the reverse.

Nursing is a hierarchical profession in which orders are followed according to rank, not sex. The nurses thus expected the nurse assistant to do what they told him. As a Nigerian male, Ikem felt that he should not have to take directions from females, despite his lower professional ranking. Unless someone with this cultural disposition can be placed under the supervision of another man, it will be difficult to maintain a viable working relationship on the floor.

Leadership

74   Problems also arise from the traditionally passive female roles valued in most Asian cultures. Myung Soon Park, a Korean charge nurse in intensive coronary care was an excellent worker. She was quiet, industrious, and knowledgeable. She gave the patients good care and was proficient in using the specialized equipment in the unit. In her role as charge nurse, however, Myung Soon was perceived as incompetent. She was unable to lead. She did not offer strong guidance to her staff. She did not counsel or reprimand them. She was indecisive and became apologetic when anyone made a mistake.

Although Myung Soon's personality was partly to blame, her submissiveness was consistent with the traditional role of Korean women. Korean culture is hierarchical, and the ideal woman is passive and subservient. She is taught to avoid conflict and maintain harmony. These values made it difficult for Myung Soon to perform the functions of a good charge nurse. Her co-workers liked her personally but were frustrated by her professional performance.

Myung Soon was aware of the problems she was having. Counseling helped her to realize she could not handle her job. She resigned as charge nurse but continued on as a staff nurse.

Doctors and Nurses

75   The subservient role of traditional Asian women is illustrated by the following incident. Janine, an Anglo nurse, and Lourdes, a Filipino nurse, were passing out patients' breakfast trays while the physicians were making rounds. One doctor grabbed a cup of coffee and a carton of milk from a tray. Lourdes rolled her eyes but said nothing. Janine told him the milk and coffee belonged to a patient. He replied that he needed it more than the patient did. Janine persisted. "If you take that, it means that patient doesn't get his morning coffee. Think how you'd feel."

As the angry physician headed down the hall, he deliberately dropped the coffee cup on the floor. Lourdes jumped to get a towel and clean up the mess. Janine stopped her, insisting that the physician clean it up himself. Lourdes looked at her in shock and replied, "You've got guts!"

Janine responded to the physician's behavior with typical American assertiveness. Filipinos are raised to respect authority. Rolling her eyes was her only visible sign of frustration. She was also trying to avoid conflict and maintain harmony, important Asian values.

76   Filipino respect for authority also helps explain why Miguela, another Filipino nurse, took the blame for something that was the

doctor's fault. A specialist physician called the intensive care nursery at 6 A.M. and spoke with Miguela. He asked why Dr. Michaels, the resident physician, had not included specific medications in a child's treatment. Miguela said she would speak to him. She passed on the specialist's recommendations, but Dr. Michaels chose not to act on them.

At the shift change, Miguela made her report to Roberta, the patient care coordinator, and the incoming nurses. Roberta questioned Dr. Michaels about the medication. Miguela interrupted, stating, "It's my fault. I should have thought of that myself. . . . I've checked the orders and the blood work results and I should have considered that." Roberta defended Miguela, saying it was not her responsibility; she had told Dr. Michaels. It had become his responsibility. The resident agreed and absolved Miguela of any blame.

Miguela later explained to Roberta that she could not let Dr. Michaels take the blame because she did not want to see him "lose face," especially in front of a nurse. The American nurse in the following situation lacked such concern for the doctor involved.

Dr. Fukushima, a Japanese physician, ordered Lisa to give a patient a certain dosage of a medication. Lisa refused on the grounds that the dosage might be harmful to the patient. Dr. Fukushima insisted, but she was adamant. The interesting twist to this situation is that when Dr. Fukushima reported Lisa to her supervisor, he suggested that she should have agreed to give the medication but simply not have done it.

Asians believe it is important both to avoid conflict and to show respect for authority. Rather than refuse directly, it is more appropriate to agree to the supervisor's face and then not follow through. Americans, in contrast, feel it is important to be direct and honest. Disagreement is not avoided. Assertiveness is valued, as is an egalitarian ideal. Dr. Fukushima's major complaint was not that the nurse disobeyed him, but that she disagreed to his face, thereby denying him proper respect.

It would be easy to suggest that nurses dealing with Asian physicians take that advice, but it is not that simple. Laws require nurses to follow through on orders they agree to. Nurses would be well-advised, however, to remember that Asian men are very concerned about their dignity and self-esteem.

Passive versus Assertive Behavior

A few examples have been given of the passive, submissive behavior of Filipino nurses. Many other nurses, however, report the complete opposite. They say that Filipino nurses can be very assertive, to the point of aggressiveness. What accounts for this discrepancy?

As in any culture, people are born with personality traits that fall along a continuum. Different cultures, however, value and reinforce different aspects of the continuum. If a child is by nature passive and the culture reinforces passivity, socialization will be easy. If the child is by nature assertive, socialization will be difficult, but possible. If when that child grows up, he or she moves to a country where assertiveness is valued, years of socialization to be passive may be suddenly undone, as that individual's true nature comes through. The assertiveness may even be exaggerated as a result of years of repression.

Thus passive Filipino nurses are the ones who were by nature passive even before being socialized in that direction. It will be very difficult to train them to be assertive. The aggressive ones are most likely those who were socialized to be passive against their inherent nature and who now have cultural (American) permission to be assertive.

Preferential Treatment

78   The gender of a child can influence the treatment it receives from the family. A fifteen-year-old Taiwanese boy named Henry Ting was dying of liver cancer. His parents spent as much time with him as possible during the year he was a patient at the hospital. One of them always spent the night with Henry, even though they had two daughters, aged eleven and thirteen, at home. Henry's mother prepared most of his meals. His father often drove to Chinatown to obtain Chinese herbs they hoped would help his condition. Mr. and Mrs. Ting were extremely devoted parents—at least to their son. The nurses were shocked to hear the Tings state on several occasions that it would have been better if one of their daughters had cancer instead. Did they value their daughters so little?

As discussed in the previous chapter, sons play an important role in traditional Chinese culture. Henry was their first-born and their only son. He would be the one to carry on the family name and care for them in their old age. If he died, whom could they rely on? Who would carry on the Ting name? Henry had always been given preferential treatment. The daughters understood their parents' attitude and did not seem to mind. It was the way things were. They, too, spent all their free time with Henry, catering to his frequent demands.

The nurses had difficulty accepting this situation. They understood the Tings' position intellectually but not emotionally. They responded by frequently pointing out how kind and sweet their daughters were. They also recommended that a psychologist meet with the family. The session was a waste of time. Although polite, the Tings

refused to speak openly with the psychologist. In Asian culture psychotherapy is reserved for the hopelessly mentally insane and carries a
great deal of stigma. It is not surprising that they would not speak with
him.

After a year in the hospital, Henry died. Two years later, his
parents had still not recovered. They visited the cemetery daily. The
elder daughter did volunteer work at the hospital to help "pay" for the
care Henry received, and the younger daughter planned to join her
when she became sixteen.

Understanding the importance of males in Chinese culture makes   79
the following case more comprehensible. A Chinese couple, the Lews,
had a two-year-old daughter named Anna and a one-year-old son
named John. John was retarded, had chronic lung disease, and was on
a respirator. Mrs. Lew spent every moment at his bedside. She bathed
him and massaged him with lotion daily. Mr. Lew visited every evening.
Mrs. Lew left Anna's birthday party early so she could rush to the
hospital for her routine visit. When a nurse asked her why she could
not take just one evening off to be with her daughter, she replied, "But
he's my son! I'd feel guilty." The Lews even considered sending Anna
to her grandmother in China so they could spend more time with John.

When the nurses did not attend John closely enough, Mrs. Lew
would complain and then apologize, saying she "shouldn't complain."
She seemed to expect them to ignore the other infants in favor of John.
Her demands and insistence on assisting in bathing John caused ten-
sion among the nurses on the unit. They were also shocked to hear
Mrs. Lew talk about sending Anna to China.

Despite John's obvious inability to care for his parents in their old
age, the traditional importance of sons outweighed the reality of the
situation. In situations such as those involving the Lews and the Tings,
nothing can be done to change the parents' attitudes. Although it may
be difficult, nurses should try to understand their point of view.

Female Purity and Modesty

In many parts of the world, female purity and modesty are major values. These can have important repercussions in a health care setting.

A twenty-three-year-old Saudi Arabian woman named Nasrin   80
Hassan was brought into the emergency room by her husband. Stephanie, the nurse on duty, introduced herself and asked Nasrin how she
could help her. Her husband, Jamal, answered that she was bleeding
and had pain in her lower abdomen. She was three months pregnant.
Stephanie told the couple that Nasrin would have to put on a patient
gown so the doctor could examine her.

Jamal refused. He would not allow Nasrin to undress, and he certainly would not permit a strange man to examine her. Stephanie and the attending doctor explained that Nasrin was probably having a miscarriage and could bleed to death if she did not receive medical attention. Their arguments were futile. Jamal abruptly left the hospital with his wife still in pain and bleeding vaginally. Later that evening, the Hassans returned. This time, Jamal consented to having his wife transferred to another hospital, where a female doctor could examine and care for her.

81   In a similar case, a twenty-eight-year-old Arab man named Abdul Nazih refused to let a male lab technician enter his wife's room to draw blood. She had just given birth. When the nurse finally convinced Abdul of the need, he reluctantly allowed the technician in the room. He took the precaution, however, of making sure Sheida was completely covered. Only her arm stuck out from beneath the blankets. Abdul watched the technician intently throughout the procedure.

Another time, the toilet in Sheida's room overflowed. Abdul flew into a rage when three men from engineering and housekeeping were about to enter the room after knocking. He refused to allow them in. The toilet went unrepaired until the couple left the next day.

All three incidents stem from the fact that among Arabs family honor is one of the highest values. Since family honor is tied to female purity, extreme modesty and sexual segregation must be maintained at all times. Hospitals that do not have female physicians on staff should have a referral system so one can be found when needed. Female housekeepers should clean the rooms of Middle Eastern females. Male nurses definitely should not be assigned to female Muslim patients. Same-sex staff should be used whenever possible.

Female Circumcision

82   An Egyptian woman in labor presented an unusual problem for the nursing staff. Her vagina was severely deformed, and they were unable to find any of the appropriate "landmarks." The entire area appeared to have been badly burned, yet no other parts of her body showed evidence of fire. The doctor and nurses were mystified. They did not realize that the woman had been circumcised.

One way female purity is maintained in the Middle East is by keeping the woman covered and veiled. Another method used in some remote regions, and particularly throughout parts of Africa, is female circumcision. Circumcision is believed to reduce the sexual desire of women. Without it, women might be unable to control their exceptionally strong libido, and family honor might be lost.

Circumcision is generally performed when a girl is seven or eight years old. Older women will come in the night, hold her down, and then start cutting. The most minor form of circumcision involves cutting off the tip of the clitoris. The most severe form, known as infibulation, is the removal of the entire clitoris, labia minora, and parts of the labia majora. The outer lips of the vagina are then held together with thorns, sutures, or a pastelike material. A small opening is left for urine and menstrual blood. The girl's legs are tied together for several weeks until she heals. As can be imagined, this practice often leads to a myriad of urinary, menstrual, and intrapartum problems.

In 1985, a world congress was held in Africa in an effort to reduce or eradicate the practice of female circumcision. Surprisingly, the greatest opposition to the elimination of the custom came not from men but from older women and young girls. The older women wanted to maintain tradition. The young girls were afraid that if they were not circumcised, they would be unable to find husbands. Circumcision is seen as the ultimate proof of purity; why would any boy marry a woman without a guarantee of her virginity?

Female Virginity

The importance of female virginity and purity are unfortunately well illustrated in the following case. Fatima, an eighteen-year-old Bedouin girl from a remote, conservative village, was brought into an American air force hospital in Saudi Arabia after she received a gunshot wound in her pelvis. She had been shot by her cousin Hamid. Her family had arranged for her to marry him, as was local custom, but she wanted nothing to do with him. She was in love with someone else. An argument ensued, and Hamid left. He returned several hours later, drunk, and shot Fatima, leaving her paralyzed from the waist down.

Fatima's parents cared for her for several weeks after the incident but finally brought her to the hospital, looking for a "magic" cure. The physician took a series of x-rays to determine the extent of Fatima's injuries. To his surprise, they revealed that she was pregnant. Sarah, the American nurse on duty, was asked to give her a pelvic exam. She confirmed the report on the x-rays. Fatima, however, had no idea that she was carrying a child. Bedouin girls are not given any sex education.

Three physicians were involved in the case: an American neurosurgeon who had worked in the region for two years; a European obstetrics and gynecology specialist who had lived in the Middle East for ten years; and a young American internist who had recently arrived. No Muslims were involved. The x-ray technician was sworn to secrecy. They all realized they had a potentially explosive situation

83

on their hands. Tribal law punished out-of-wedlock pregnancies with death.

The obstetrician arranged to have Fatima flown to London for a secret abortion. He told the family that the bullet wound was complicated and required the technical skill available in a British hospital.

The only opposition came from the American internist. He felt the family should be told about the girl's condition. The other two physicians explained the seriousness of the situation to him. Girls in Fatima's condition were commonly stoned to death. An out-of-wedlock pregnancy is seen as a direct slur upon the males of the family, particularly the father and brothers, who are charged with protecting her honor. Her misconduct implies that the males did not do their duty. The only way for the family to regain honor is to punish the girl—by death.

Finally, the internist acquiesced and agreed to say nothing. At the last minute, however, the reluctant physician decided he could not live with his conscience. As Fatima was being wheeled to the waiting airplane, he told her father about her pregnancy.

The father did not say a word. He simply grabbed his daughter off the gurney, threw her into the car, and drove away. Two weeks later, the obstetrician saw one of Fatima's brothers. He asked him how Fatima was. The boy looked down at the ground and mumbled, "She died." Family honor had been restored. The ethnocentric internist had a nervous breakdown and had to be sent back to the United States.

Modesty

84   Modesty is important in many cultures, and not just for women. A Gypsy king was hospitalized with pneumonia. The staff found it very difficult to treat him because of the restrictions he imposed. The nurses were not allowed to bathe him, and not even the male physician was allowed to examine him below the waist.

Sexual segregation is observed in Gypsy culture and may help explain why the king would not allow female nurses to bathe him. The area below the waist is considered *marime* (dirty) and calls for extreme modesty in both men and women. In such cases, same-sex nurses and physicians are advisable, and examinations below the waist should be approached cautiously and with explanations regarding their necessity.

85   Modesty is valued in Asian cultures as well. Phan Tran, a fifty-seven-year-old Vietnamese woman, was brought into the emergency room by her husband, son, and daughter-in-law. Mrs. Tran had not

been eating well for the past month and her fluid intake was poor. A stroke two years earlier had left her paralyzed on the left side. She was rapidly deteriorating, and her family was concerned. The information was conveyed by her son; Mrs. Tran spoke no English.

After examining her, the doctor ordered some tests, along with a Foley catheter and intravenous therapy. Even though she was covered from the waist up, Mrs. Tran was extremely embarrassed when the nurse inserted the catheter. She avoided eye contact and turned her face to the wall. The nurse, sensing her discomfort, did the procedure as quickly as possible.

The area between the waist and knees is considered particularly private by Southeast Asians. Even though Mrs. Tran's upper body was covered, the most intimate part was being exposed. Traditional Asian physicians do not touch a woman's body except to take her pulse. Instead, the woman points to the corresponding area of a doll to indicate the site of her problem. Only a woman's husband should see her genitals.

There is little to be done in such cases other than to respect the patient's modesty and to keep as much of her body covered as possible. Only procedures that are absolutely necessary should be done. Routine pelvic exams, for example, should be avoided.

Sofia Toledo, a sixty-five-year-old upper-class Mexican woman, refused to be dialyzed when she learned that her usual dialysis station was unavailable. She said she would wait until her next treatment, when she could have her customary place. Unfortunately, this was not a viable alternative. Missing a treatment could result in serious complications or even death. When Julia, the nurse, asked her why the new station was unacceptable, Mrs. Toledo was very vague.

Julia finally called Mrs. Toledo's daughter, and together they solved the problem. Mrs. Toledo's usual station was unusual in that it could not be seen very well by the nurses or the patients at the other dialysis stations. The rest of the stations were very open, designed for high visibility by the nurses. To be dialyzed, the patient had to remove her pants and don a patient gown. Her underwear was exposed during the process. Mrs. Toledo's sense of modesty, a quality very strong in Hispanic women, made the more open station intolerable.

Julia said that at the time she found Mrs. Toledo's behavior annoying. She and the other nurses saw it as a delay that would prevent them from leaving early. They did not want to have the extra work of moving machinery or remixing the dialysate. She did not understand the importance of modesty in Hispanic culture, but she did realize that it was important to Mrs. Toledo, a normally compliant patient. In this case, a screen or curtain might have alleviated the problem.

86

Summary

What conclusions can be drawn from these cases? In general, same-sex physicians and nurses should be assigned if possible when dealing with non-Anglo ethnic groups. Try to keep patients' genitals covered whenever possible. Recognize that sex roles and authority figures vary, though males generally hold the dominant position. Use that knowledge when dealing with patients or families from other ethnic groups. This advice may rankle many women, who may interpret it as reinforcing male domination. Perhaps it does, but if the goals are patient compliance, smooth working relationships, and the best possible patient care, this will be the most expedient way of achieving them.

Chapter 6

Birth

Increasingly, people enter the world in a hospital. Birth is an emotional and generally painful occasion imbued with cultural ritual—and thus, once again, we find the potential for misunderstanding and conflict.

Preparation

Confusion can begin before a woman enters the labor and delivery rooms. In one case, a nurse named Judith came to "prep" an Iranian woman and was surprised to find her pubic area already completely shaved. American women are usually uncomfortable about being shaved in the pubic area and require constant reassurance that more hair is not being shaved off than necessary. For this reason, nurses pride themselves on shaving off the minimal amount of pubic hair necessary for delivery.

Jasmine, an Americanized Iranian woman, later explained to Judith that many Iranian women completely shave their bodies in preparation for both their wedding night and the birth of their children. Although Jasmine did not know the reason for this custom, she thought it might be because Persian women are generally very hairy and shaving might reduce their embarrassment about it.

Judith reflected upon her own discomfort when others saw her normally clean-shaven legs covered with stubble. She also realized that the Iranian practice made her job easier. These two thoughts helped her view the situation with cultural relativism rather than with ethnocentrism.

Sometimes fears stem from a lack of information. Lottie, a preg- nant Black woman from the Deep South, came into the labor and delivery area extremely upset. Her membranes had ruptured, and she feared this would mean a difficult and dry birth. Actually, the body continues to produce amniotic fluid until delivery. Lottie, however, did not know this. Instead she believed that her early loss of fluid would result in a lack of fluid during delivery.

In a case such as this, a recital of the facts will often calm the patient. In this particular situation, Lottie provided her own solution by drinking two bottles of mineral oil in between contractions. She thought that the slippery properties of the oil would lubricate the birth canal and help the baby to slide out more easily. This response is consistent with the rich tradition of folk remedies found in the American Black culture, in which it is believed that nature provides a cure for every ailment.

Labor

89   A labor and delivery team faced a difficult problem with a patient from Southwest Africa. Despite repeated requests, Grace refused to push. Her mother had raised her to believe that a woman dies eight times during labor. Feeling herself on the verge of her eighth death, Grace feared that if she pushed again, she would die her final death. Unfortunately, her doctor could not convince Grace otherwise and decided to perform a cesarean section.

Labor Pains

Individuals respond differently to pain, although cultural norms often dictate how it is expressed. This holds true for the pains of labor.

90   Doris, a Black American, and Miguela, a Filipino, were delivering their babies at the same time. Miguela's contractions were very strong and closely spaced. The baby was positioned a little too high, and there was some discussion of a possible c-section. Despite her difficulties, Miguela cooperated with the doctor's instructions and labored in silence. The only signs of pain or discomfort were her look of concentration and her white knuckles.

In contrast, Doris lay in the delivery room across the hall, moaning and groaning. Although the delivery was progressing normally, her cries increased in intensity. Finally, her blood-curdling yells resounded through the halls. The hospital personnel compared Doris's behavior to Miguela's and naturally rated it unfavorably. Why was Doris acting like such a baby? Why couldn't she control herself as Miguela did?

Cultural differences account for the behavioral differences. Miguela's culture values stoicism; Doris's culture does not. Filipinos believe that a woman must experience pain and discomfort as a part of childbirth. To express these feelings, however, brings shame upon her. This is true in most Asian cultures.

The culture of American Blacks does not place such restrictions upon its women. Varied emotional expression has always been a part of Black culture. Doris was culturally normal in expressing her pain. Another Black woman might have suffered in silence and still have been culturally normal.

Mexican women are notorious for loud behavior during labor and delivery. It is often possible to identify a Mexican woman in labor simply from the "aye yie yies" emanating from her room. Although this chant can be annoying to nurses and patients alike, it is actually a form of "folk Lamaze." To repeat "aye yie yie" several times in succession requires long, slow, deep breaths. "Aye yie yie" is not just an expression of pain; it is a culturally appropriate method of *relieving* pain.

Middle Eastern women also tend to be very expressive during labor. Pasha, an Arab woman, let out a yell with each contraction. Even though she had an intravenous line, an internal fetal monitor, and a monitor to measure uterine contractions, she began to writhe all over the bed in pain. Her doctor spoke to her in Arabic but could not calm her down. Pasha's labor lasted many hours. Twice the obstetrician tried and failed to administer an epidural, primarily because she would not lie still. Fortunately, Pasha finally arrived at the transition stage and delivered.

Although her behavior may have appeared excessive to observers, it was fully consistent with traditional Arab culture. Women are expected to express their pain loudly; generally this brings about a more caring response from those assisting in the delivery. Out of cultural context, however, Pasha's behavior had the opposite effect. The staff became impatient, and many nurses avoided Pasha's room unless it was absolutely necessary to attend her. American nurses value cooperation; a cooperative patient is one who is stoic and follows directions. Uncooperative patients, like Pasha, are often avoided.

Women from some cultures may profit greatly from emphasizing their pain during childbirth. A labor and delivery nurse reported that the most difficult patient she ever attended was Robabeh, an Iranian woman, who yelled and screamed for the entire duration of her labor. After she delivered their child, Robabeh's husband presented her with a three-karat diamond ring. When her nurse commented on the expensive gift, Robabeh responded dramatically, "Of course. He made me suffer so much!" Iranian custom is to compensate a woman for her suffering during childbirth by giving her gifts. The greater the suffering, the more expensive the gifts she will receive, especially if she delivers a boy. Her cries indicate how much she is suffering.

How can hospital personnel deal with the variety of expressions of women's pain during labor and delivery? As one nurse put it, there are techniques for controlling pain that are more effective than yelling, but the delivery table is hardly the place to educate women in coping skills. If nurses understand why patients behave the way they do, however, they can be more supportive.

As for the patients themselves, it might be very disconcerting for an Asian woman accustomed to controlling her emotions to labor next to a highly expressive Mexican or Middle Eastern woman. Ideally, women might be placed in rooms with women from cultures similar to theirs. Unfortunately, this is not always possible.

Labor Attendants

It is currently standard American practice for a woman's husband to assist her in labor and in the delivery of their child. Husbands are expected to be helpful and to attend to their wives' needs. Unfortunately, things do not always work out this way.

93   Naomi, an Orthodox Jewish woman, was in labor with her third child. She had severe pains, which were alleviated only by back rubs between contractions. Her husband, Aaron, asked Marge, a nurse, to remain in the room to rub Naomi's back. Because she had two other patients to care for, Marge began to instruct Aaron on how to massage his wife. To Marge's surprise, he immediately interrupted her, explaining that he could not touch his wife because she was unclean. Marge, assuming he meant Naomi was sweaty from labor, suggested that he massage her through the sheets. In an annoyed tone, Aaron again explained that he could not touch his wife because she was unclean. He then left the room.

Marge later learned from Naomi that "unclean" referred to a spiritual, rather than a physical, condition. According to the Orthodox Jewish tradition, the blood of both menstruation and birth render a woman unclean and her husband is forbidden to touch her during those times.

Labor and delivery nurses must do everything for the Orthodox Jewish patient whose husband will not participate. This often generates resentment toward both the patient and her husband. Nurses sometimes try to avoid being assigned to Orthodox patients or assign another Jewish nurse to attend to them. As always, a good solution is education. If nurses understand why an Orthodox husband cannot get involved in his wife's labor, they may be more accepting.

94   An Arab husband can be similarly unhelpful during his wife's labor and delivery. After his wife, Azar, was admitted to the unit, Ahmed told the nurse that he would wait outside. Realizing that her patient did not speak English, she asked Ahmed to stay and act as

translator. At first, he refused, insisting that it was a woman's placc to help in birthing, not a man's. Since there were no Arab women available to translate, however, he reluctantly agreed to stay.

During her entire labor, Ahmed ignored Azar except to translate as requested. She was obviously having a difficult time, expressing her pain quite loudly, but he did nothing to comfort her. The staff grew angry with him. It was inadvisable to insist that Ahmed stay with Azar during childbirth. Because it was inappropriate for him to be there, he felt extremely uncomfortable and did little to help her situation.

A similar case involved a young Mexican couple. Judging from her "aye yie yies," Juanita was in a great deal of pain. When the nurse insisted that her husband, Carlos, attend to her, he very reluctantly entered the room. Rather than help soothe Juanita by holding her hand, speaking gently to her, or wiping her brow, he stood in the corner. He looked up, down, everywhere but at her. The nurse became very angry. She felt that because Carlos had gotten Juanita into this position in the first place, he should be willing to comfort her.

In another instance, a Mexican woman named Carmelita had recently moved to California. She was five months pregnant when she began to bleed vaginally. Her mother and husband brought her to the emergency room, and it became clear that a premature delivery was inevitable. Labor lasted one and a half hours. During this time, Carmelita continuously cried out for her mother. The nursing staff brought her husband into the room to provide moral support, but Carmelita ignored him. He, in turn, sat in a chair a few feet from her bed with his back to her and stared out the door. Carmelita continued to cry for her mother.

In Mexico, it is inappropriate for a husband to attend his wife during delivery. It is a woman's job—ideally the job of her mother. This may be related to the extreme modesty of Mexican women. Whatever the reason, cultural tradition dictates that a husband not see his wife or child until the delivery is over and both have been cleaned and dressed.

For those who find these cultural practices hard to understand, consider suddenly being forced to watch one's parents havc scx. How would we feel? Would we stand there and coach them? Wipe their sweaty brows? Or would we stand in a corner, looking up, down, everywhere but at them? Sexual relations occur in the presence of children in some parts of the world but are taboo in American culture, just as it is taboo for a Mexican man to watch his wife give birth, though it is a common practice for American men. Younger, more Americanized Mexican couples may want to participate in the delivery process together, but it should not be assumed that the husband is the proper person to coach his wife in this situation.

In the case of the Mexican woman who delivered prematurely, the doctor and nurses involved judged the patient as immature and her husband as unsupportive and ineffective. One of the nurses later suggested that the staff purposely excluded the patient's mother from the delivery room to punish Carmelita for her "immature, inappropriate" behavior. Since the rules allowed only one visitor at a time, the husband's presence prevented Carmelita's mother from attending her daughter. The nurses apparently felt it was her husband's job, and he would attend her or no one would.

In general, Hispanic women prefer that their mothers attend them in labor. This is also true of Asian women, although sometimes the mother-in-law is considered more appropriate. Traditionally, a Chinese couple resides with the husband's parents, and the daughter-in-law spends much of her married life taking care of the needs of her in-laws. This is reversed during childbirth. Then, a mother-in-law must attend to the needs of her daughter-in-law, both during delivery and throughout the monthlong lying-in period.

Postpartum Lying-in Period

97   Mei-Li, a Chinese woman in her mid-twenties, had just given birth. The hospital staff became concerned when she would neither eat the hospital food nor bathe. Her only nourishment came from the food brought in by her family. Later Mei-Li explained that custom prevented her from bathing for seven days after childbirth and permitted her to eat only certain foods.

98   The following cases also illustrate how Asian cultural practices may result in behavior regarded as odd or unhealthy by Westerners. A twenty-eight-year-old Vietnamese woman named Hanh Ly gave birth to her first child by cesarean section. After the delivery, she requested ice water. Her mother emphatically refused, insisting that she be given hot water to drink instead. After a discussion in Vietnamese, the patient compromised and asked for a pitcher of warm water. The nurse noted that despite the warm temperature, Hanh Ly wore socks and spread a robe over the sheets. When asked if she was cold, she said no.

99   Su Yong, a nineteen-year-old Vietnamese woman, returned to the hospital with a high fever and abdominal pain twelve days after giving birth. During her stay, she rejected most of the food and liquids prepared by the hospital, refused to shower or wash her hair (despite increasingly strong body odor), and would not get out of bed except to use the bathroom. When she insisted on mounds of blankets despite her high temperature and sweating, the nurses feared for her health.

A thirty-four-year-old Filipino woman named Flores gave birth via 100 c-section. On the following day, her nurse prepared to bathe her, but she refused. The day after that, the nurse brought Flores a basin of water and a sponge so she could bathe herself. Several hours later, the water was still clean and the towels untouched. When questioned, Flores explained that it was the custom in her culture to refrain from bathing or showering for ten days after giving birth.

The patients described above were all practicing versions of the traditional lying-in period observed throughout much of Asia and Latin America. For a period of time after a woman gives birth, her body is thought to be weak and especially susceptible to outside forces. The new mother is encouraged to avoid both exercise and bathing. These traditional practices come into direct conflict with Western health care, which promotes exercise and bathing for new mothers as soon as possible following childbirth.

The traditional practice in China is called "doing the month." It is important to keep the room warm, lest cold or wind enter the new mother's joints. Bathing is considered dangerous for similar reasons. No matter how hot the weather, the traditional Chinese woman will want the windows closed and the air conditioning off.

In Asia, health is believed to depend upon keeping the body in a state of balance. Pregnancy is generally thought to be a hot condition. Giving birth causes the sudden loss of yang, or heat, which must be restored. The most effective way to do this is to eat yang foods, such as chicken. Cold liquids should be avoided lest the system receive too great a shock.

Traditional Asian thought has it that the price for not "doing the month" is aches, pains, arthritis, and other ailments when one is old. Although practical circumstances may prevent a woman from observing the entire month, many want to practice at least a shortened version of it. This explains why the patients in the cases described above refused ice water in preference for hot, rejected bathing or exercise, insisted upon keeping extremely warm, and ate only certain foods.

In Mexico the lying-in period lasts for six weeks, the time believed necessary for the womb to return to normal. (In fact, forty-two days is generally the amount of time it takes for the uterus to return to its prepregnant size.) The customs involved are essentially identical to those of the Asian practice: the woman is to rest, stay very warm, and avoid bathing and exercise. Special foods designed to restore warmth to the body are prescribed. Disregarding these practices is believed to lead to aches and pains in later life.

The custom of lying-in explains why a twenty-six-year-old Mexi- 101 can mother did not accompany her husband and two children to the hospital to visit her premature newborn. The baby girl, who had been born ten weeks early, was given an excellent chance for survival. The hospital had a policy of family-centered care and encouraged early visitation and touching of the infant. The nurses were concerned in this case about maternal-infant bonding. They did not understand that the patient was practicing the traditional lying-in period and could not do anything other than rest in bed. Had the nurses known this, they might have sent photographs of the baby home to the mother and encouraged her to call for progress reports.

There are three additional points to be made about the lying-in period. First, it is designed to give a woman a period of rest between childbirth and returning to work. The women who practice this custom are usually Asian and Latin American. In these cultures women traditionally did not return to office work, but to physical labor in the fields. Because they usually had large families, it might be the only time they had to rest.

Second, avoidance of bathing may also have practical origins. In many countries the water is impure and filled with harmful bacteria. Bathing could introduce these organisms into the body and cause illness. Although conditions in the United States are different, the custom continues.

The third point involves the ways in which different generations adhere to customs. As with Hanh Ly, the Vietnamese woman who wanted ice water but was advised by her mother to drink hot water instead, daughters may be less interested in following traditional customs than their mothers. To avoid her mother's nagging, the daughter may comply with the cultural traditions when the mother is present. When the patient is alone, a nurse may suggest bathing, exercise, and so forth.

Compromises can be made. Although it is important for a patient to drink fluids after childbirth, both hot tea and hot water with lemon deliver the same amount of liquid as ice water without violating custom. Using boiled water (cooled down) may make a sponge bath more acceptable. (This was done in China to remove impurities.) The patient should be kept covered and given socks or slippers to walk in. It is important to explain the reason for bathing and exercise and not to assume that the patient will follow orders that violate the traditions and wisdom of her own culture.

Bonding

102

Maternal-infant bonding has become a major concern of Western health care professionals in recent decades. Poor bonding has been

associated with failure to thrive, child abuse, and psychological problems. It is therefore not surprising that doctors and nurses become
concerned when they observe cultural beliefs and practices that appear
to reflect poor bonding. They often do not. An example is the case of
Thanh Vo, a Vietnamese woman who came to the hospital to deliver
her fifth child. After giving birth to a son, she refused to cuddle him,
although she willingly provided minimal care such as feeding and
changing his diaper. The nursery nurse, feeling sorry for the "neglected" baby, picked him up, cuddled him, and stroked the top of his
head. Mrs. Vo and her husband became visibly upset. The baby, who
had jaundice, had to remain in the hospital for several days after Mrs.
Vo went home. She did not visit her baby even once during the time he
remained in the hospital.

In the past, nurses who worked in areas with a large Vietnamese
population often referred these mothers to social services. Eventually,
however, they came to understand that the apparently neglectful behavior did not reflect poor bonding, but instead indicated cultural
belief and traditions.

Many people in the more rural areas of Vietnam believe in spirits.
Since spirits are particularly attracted to infants and likely to "steal"
them (by inducing death), it is important that parents do everything
possible to avoid attracting attention to their newborn. For this reason,
infants are not verbally fussed over. They are sometimes even dressed
in old clothes to "fool" the spirits. The apparent lack of interest new
parents demonstrate reflects an intense love and concern for the child,
rather than the opposite.

Mrs. Vo and her husband were probably distressed over the nurse's
attention to their baby for two reasons. First, they may have feared having attention drawn to their baby. Second, Southeast Asians view the
head as private and personal. It is also seen as the seat of the soul and is
not to be touched. Not only did the nurse risk attracting the attention of
dangerous spirits, but she also stroked the child in a taboo area.

Why did Mrs. Vo not come to visit her son in the hospital after she
was discharged? She was probably practicing lying-in and was at home
resting while her internal organs resumed their normal position in her
body.

Another Vietnamese tradition that is often mistakenly interpreted
by Western medical personnel as a sign of poor bonding is a delay in
naming the child. A newborn's name is often decided upon by the
family in a naming ceremony that takes place in the parents' house with
relatives present. Failing to name the child in the hospital does not
reflect a lack of interest in the child. It is adherence to a custom that
emphasizes the child's importance as a member of the family.

Nurses can best deal with Vietnamese mothers by following their lead. If the parents do not fuss over the child, nurses should not either. In any event, they should avoid touching the infant's head. And as long as a mother can feed and hold her baby properly, they should not be concerned about an apparent lack of interest. It is merely an illusion.

103   Nurses were similarly disturbed when an East Indian mother refused to hold her baby except to feed her. The nurses' concerns were quieted, however, when they later learned that the only care many Indian new mothers provide for their infants is to nurse them. A family member takes over its other care. In a variant of the lying-in period common throughout Asia and Latin America, the new mother is encouraged to rest in bed and eat a special diet including large amounts of milk, cooked butter, ghee (clarified butter), and high-protein foods.

104   In another example of the lying-in period, an East Indian woman, a Sikh, created a difficult situation for the nurses and her roommate. After delivering her baby, she lay in bed doing nothing. She was constantly surrounded by female relatives who did everything for her. The nurses even had to carry her to the bathroom because she refused to get up to urinate.

During a staff conference on this patient, one of the nurses suggested putting her in a room with Rapinder, another Indian patient, who might be tolerant about the constant stream of visitors. An Indian nurse on staff quickly pointed out that Rapinder was Hindu. Hindus and Sikhs do not always get along, and it would be unwise to assign them to the same room. The fact that two people are from the same country does not guarantee that they share the same culture.

Rejection

105   Occasionally parents will reject a newborn. Such was the case with a Middle Eastern couple after the wife, Salomi, gave birth to a baby girl. At the moment of delivery, while the doctor and nurses were oohing and aahing over the infant, her father turned and abruptly left the delivery room. Salomi herself would not hold or even look at her child. When a nurse approached the lobby where many of the woman's relatives had earlier been anxiously awaiting the birth, she found that they had all left. Later, Salomi held her child, but she refused to lavish any loving attention upon her.

The nurse who reported this incident could not understand why parents would respond so negatively to such a joyous event. A Middle Eastern acquaintance later told her the reason. Salomi and her husband had two daughters but no sons. Males are extremely important in Middle Eastern culture because they carry on the family name and all wealth is passed on through them. Many groups trace descent through the male line only, unlike our own system, which recognizes both the mother's and father's sides of the family. Even in groups that have adopted more Western patterns of inheritance, the traditional importance of the male may remain. For Salomi and her husband, a third daughter was a great disappointment.

There is little that the staff can do in such a situation, other than refer the parents to social services. Parents will rarely change ideas that have years of cultural tradition behind them. The important thing for nurses to do is to watch for signs of neglect.

Baby Care

In yet another case, a nurse attempted to explain baby care techniques to Middle Eastern parents. Since the new mother was not feeling well, the nurse began to explain everything to her husband. To the nurse's surprise, he refused to listen, stating that in his country men did not get involved in child care; it was a woman's job. Although economic and other factors may intervene, there is generally a very strict delineation of sex roles in the Middle East. Childrearing is a woman's responsibility. A man deals with his children later on in their lives. In such situations, it may be best to wait until a new mother is well enough to listen to instructions rather than try to explain things to her husband.

106

Breastfeeding

It is well known that the colostrum that fills a new mother's breasts before her milk comes in is rich in antibodies that fight infections to which newborns might be subject. Western doctors and nurses emphasize the importance of feeding infants colostrum. Many ethnic groups, however, refuse to do so.

Sofia Lopez, a Mexican-American, gave birth to a son. The nurse wheeled the baby into Sofia's room and handed him to her to be nursed. Instead, Sofia pointed to her breasts and said, "*No leche, no leche*" (No milk, no milk). Pedro, her husband, explained to the nurse that Sofia would bottle-feed now and breastfeed when she returned home.

107

According to the nurse who related this example, most of the Mexican women who gave birth in a hospital near the Mexican border followed the same pattern—early bottle-feeding, later breastfeeding. Because colostrum is so important, this practice worries health care professionals.

Many Mexican women believe they have no milk until their breasts enlarge and they can actually see it. Some perceive colostrum as "bad milk" or "spoiled" and thus not good for a baby. Many do not realize that milk production is stimulated by nursing. Still others are very modest and are embarrassed to expose their breasts while nursing in the hospital.

The best way to deal with this situation is through education. Explain the importance of colostrum to the baby's health. If the mother's concern is to provide "real" milk for the baby, tell her that nursing on the colostrum will help it to come more quickly. The new mother should also be given privacy while nursing her infant.

Similar advice could be given to the Vietnamese mother who refused to breastfeed in the hospital, explaining that she would do so when she returned home. The Vietnamese also believe that colostrum is dirty and often delay nursing until after their milk comes in.

Belly Buttons

108   American medical professionals fear germs. For this reason, they are almost obsessively concerned with cleanliness. A Mexican custom designed to create an attractive belly button is thus likely to disturb them. A coin is applied to an infant's navel and the area is wrapped tightly with a cloth to keep the coin in place. Sometimes the job of keeping the navel flat is left entirely to the belly band. In any case, a protruding belly button is considered unsightly. Loving mothers will do what they can to ensure that their babies are attractive.

Health care professionals are concerned about the possibility of infection from a dirty cloth or coin. To respect their tradition and address health concerns, Mexican mothers should be taught the importance of using clean cloths and wiping the coin with alcohol before putting it on the baby's body. Most mothers are willing to make the minor adjustments necessary to ensure the health of their children.

Birth Control

A chapter on birth must also acknowledge efforts to prevent the event. As one nurse learned, discussions of birth control practices can have unexpected results when cultural factors are not taken into account.

109   Connie was a nurse-instructor in a postnatal education program that covered a variety of topics from personal hygiene and child care to birth control. All of the fifteen women attending were of Mexican descent. Most were new to the United States and spoke no English. Connie made her presentations in Spanish. The last class covered birth

control, and the women were asked to bring their husbands to this session.

Soon after the session started, many of the women began to blush and lower their heads. Some of the men got up and left the room; others moved to the back where they stood against the wall. The few men who remained in their seats appeared extremely uncomfortable. Connie noticed what was happening, but she had no idea what to do about it. She decided to ignore it and continue her presentation. When she finished, everyone left the room, quickly and quietly.

Why did the people react so negatively? Most Mexicans are Catholic, and birth control methods other than rhythm are unacceptable. Not only was Connie discussing other methods, she was advocating their use.

Even if religious prohibitions were not an issue, specific methods may have been. Condoms are generally associated with prostitutes. To suggest that a man use a condom with his wife is, in a sense, insulting her. Diaphragms may not be the best choice for women who are very modest, as Mexican women tend to be. They may not be comfortable touching themselves "down there" in order to insert and remove a diaphragm. Modesty may also contraindicate an IUD because it may be embarrassing to have a male physician insert it. Perhaps a female gynecologist might ease this situation somewhat. Modesty may have also been partially responsible for the women's embarrassment while Connie discussed issues related to sex in mixed company.

Machismo is also at issue here. For most Latin males, children are proof of virility. An American man's status is in large part derived from the amount of money he earns, whereas a Mexican man's status is derived primarily from the number of children he sires. To suggest that a Mexican man limit the number of children he produces is akin to encouraging an American man to limit his income. It is a suggestion not likely to be taken well and probably contributed to the reaction of many of the men attending the class.

It is also possible that talk of birth control was perceived as a form of racial genocide. It might have been better to discuss "family planning" or "spacing" children.

When giving information on birth control, it is extremely important to give clear and complete instructions on its use. One nurse related the case of an angry Mexican woman who became pregnant even though she faithfully took her birth control pill every day. Questioning revealed that the woman had inserted the pills into her vagina. Her action may have seemed logical to her; unfortunately, it was not effective.

110

111   Another Mexican woman became pregnant while using contraceptive foam. Although the failure rate with foam is much higher than with birth control pills, that was not the cause of her pregnancy. No one had explained to her how to use the foam. Since the directions on the can were in English, which she did not understand, she and her husband did what made sense to them—they applied the foam to his penis before he inserted it into her vagina.

Sterilization

Limiting the number of children is an extremely complicated issue in many cultures. Often, women and men take different positions on the issue, particularly in cultures where women have the primary responsibility for raising the children and men's major access to status and prestige is through the number of children they sire. Although a woman's status in such cultures may also derive from her role as a mother, women generally take the more practical stance.

112   Carmen, a twenty-four-year-old Mexican woman, was ready to deliver her sixth child in six years. She begged her obstetrician to perform a tubal ligation after the delivery. Hospital policy, however, required Carmen's husband to sign a consent form for the procedure, and he would not allow it. Carmen was concerned that they would not be able to feed another child; she was not even sure they could feed this one. But her husband wanted as many children as Carmen could give him. She begged the physician to tie her tubes and not tell her husband.

He refused. The hospital had been sued by women who had been sterilized at their own request. The husband would learn later that his wife had had a tubal ligation. Rather than admit it had been done at her insistence and risk losing her husband, she would claim that she had not known what she was signing or had been coerced. For this reason, many hospitals now refuse to sterilize women without their husband's consent. (Interestingly, few, if any, hospitals, require the wife's consent for a vasectomy.)

113   A forty-five-year-old Mexican woman named Luna Ortiz was advised by her obstetrician that another pregnancy might prove fatal. Her eighth pregnancy (and third cesarean) had caused a thinning of her uterine wall. Rather than have her tubes tied while she was in the hospital, Luna said she would have to discuss the matter with her husband. "He will decide what to do." Unlike Carmen, Mrs. Ortiz accepted the authority of the male to make all major decisions, including whether to have more children, regardless of how it affected her health.

A final case involves Lotty Parker, a forty-three-year-old Black woman, pregnant with her twelfth child. During a prenatal exam, the obstetrics resident asked if she had considered having her tubes tied at the time of delivery. Mrs. Parker immediately became angry, saying, "I ain't gonna have no white doctor messin' with my insides!" The resident may have felt that it was his responsibility to explain increased pregnancy risks after forty, but the Black woman apparently viewed his suggestion as a form of racial genocide. Health care personnel must be especially sensitive to this issue when dealing with patients from minority ethnic groups.

Summary

Different cultures have different traditions regarding the process of birth. Some cultures dictate that a woman suffer the pains of labor in silence; others encourage her to express or even exaggerate her pain. The birth may be attended by the husband, mother, or mother-in-law. Some cultures have postpartum rituals that a new mother must observe which contradict the recommendations of Western medical science. Some bathe and exercise as soon as possible, while others are taught to lie in bed and avoid showering and physical activity. Although immediate breastfeeding is now encouraged by doctors, women in some cultures believe it is necessary to wait several days lest the "dirty" antibody-rich colostrum harm their child. Finally, many cultures do not share our advocacy of birth control, in part because children are a major source of self-esteem for those who would otherwise have no access to status.

Some of these differences affect the health of the mother or child but others do not. Health care professionals must learn to recognize the difference. Detailed explanations and compromise are necessary when good health is the issue; cultural relativism must be exercised when it is not.

Chapter 7
Folk Medicine—Practices and Perspectives

One source of misunderstanding in the hospital stems from the practice of various folk treatments. Some can result in misdiagnosis; others
simply contradict scientific medicine. Misunderstandings can also arise
from patients' beliefs about what constitutes proper medical treatment.
Such beliefs and practices are the focus of the first part of this chapter.

A second topic concerns the concept of body image. The ideal
image varies considerably from culture to culture and may affect patients' attitudes toward specific treatments.

Coin Rubbing

A thirty-eight-year-old Cambodian male was brought into the hospital,
semicomatose, with rows of red marks on his body. He was suffering
from severe headache, nausea, vomiting, and lethargy. Once he was
hospitalized, one of his relatives began to rub the marks on his skin
with something that looked like oil.

115

The adult children of a Vietnamese woman rushed their mother
to the hospital. The emergency room personnel discovered dark red
welts running up her arms, shoulders, and chest, yet her only presenting complaint was dizziness. When questioned, her son explained that
he had rubbed her body with a quarter.

116

A nurse became concerned when she found an elderly Chinese
patient rubbing himself with a quarter; she thought he was trying to
hurt himself. When she took the coin away from him, he became very
upset, grabbed it back from her, and continued to rub his arms and
legs, leaving dark red scratches.

117

In each case, the nurses responded with a combination of disbelief, disgust, curiosity, ridicule, intolerance, and finally attempts to understand. In each case, the explanation was the same. The patients were practicing a traditional Asian form of healing known as coin rubbing. There are several variations, including heating the coin or putting oil on it, but they all involve vigorously rubbing the body with a coin. This produces red welts on the affected area, which can distract health professionals from the real problem or be mistaken for child abuse.

Underlying this practice is the belief that the illness in the body needs to be drawn out. Rubbing the body with a coin produces a raised red area, giving the appearance that the illness has been brought to the surface of the skin. It is believed that red marks will appear only on people who are ill, which is seen as further support for the effectiveness of the technique. Many Asian-Americans claim that they still practice coin rubbing because it brings relief from colds and other ailments.

118   Lack of knowledge of this widespread practice can have disastrous results. A Korean man named Sung Kim was brought into the emergency room, unconscious. His chest was covered with red welts. The family did not speak English, and there was no interpreter available. The staff assumed that Mr. Kim's lack of consciousness was related to the red welts, that both were symptoms of the same condition. They were not. Unfortunately, by the time they discovered what Mr. Kim was suffering from, it was too late to save him. Had they known to ignore the welts, they might have saved his life.

119   A Vietnamese girl named Kathy Nguyen was in her first year at an American elementary school. She was not feeling very well one morning so her mother rubbed the back of her neck with a coin. She then felt well enough to attend school. Later in the day, however, she began to feel worse and went to see the school nurse. When the nurse discovered the welts on Kathy's neck, she immediately assumed she was seeing a case of child abuse and conscientiously reported the Nguyens to the authorities. The situation was finally straightened out, but it created a great deal of needless embarrassment for Kathy's family.

It is not that Asians never abuse their children, but rubbing them with coins is not the way they do it, any more than Americans abuse their children by having thin pieces of metal wrapped around their teeth and tightened until their teeth move out of place. Braces are usually applied for merely aesthetic reasons. Coin rubbing, at least, is an attempt to heal. Apparently, it often works; only the failures show up in the medical system.

It is important that health care professionals become familiar with the practice, lest they become distracted from the real problem or mistakenly make accusations of child abuse. When such welts are observed, if the patient and family do not speak English, it would be a good idea to pull out a coin and mime rubbing the body with it. That, along with a questioning look, would probably convey the message. If the patient or family nods in agreement, the marks should be ignored.

Cupping

Another healing method that produces similarly misleading results is cupping. John Bagdasarian, a forty-six-year-old Armenian, was brought into the critical care unit with a diagnosis of acute myocardial infarction (heart attack). While doing a physical assessment, the nurse found round red marks all over his upper back which looked like burns. The staff speculated about the source of the marks. Theories ranged from birthmarks to some form of torture or sadism. An Armenian physician finally cleared up the mystery. The marks were a result of cupping.

120

The patient's family had tried to cure him of his chest pains by heating a glass and placing it on his body. The vacuum created under the glass caused the skin to rise and left the red marks. What did the Bagdasarians hope to accomplish with this procedure? Possibly they believed that John's pain was caused by cold air entering his chest. Applying a hot glass on the back is thought to equalize the imbalance in the body. Another possibility is that it was done to chase out the evil spirit that was causing the pain. In any case, when cupping did not stop the chest pains, his family brought him to the hospital.

Cupping is said to be particularly successful for treating sore muscles and is frequently practiced for that purpose in many parts of the world, including Asia, Latin America, and parts of Europe, and is taught in acupuncture colleges in the United States. As with coin rubbing, however, cupping can easily be misinterpreted by health care professionals who are not aware of the practice.

Fevers

Current medical wisdom has it that the most effective way to reduce fever is to cool the body. This is done by removing regular blankets and placing an "ice blanket" under the patient. In contrast, many cultures believe that the best way to treat a high temperature is to sweat it out. These conflicting theories are the source of another common cultural conflict in the hospital.

Hiroshi Tomita, a Japanese businessman on a trip to the United States, was admitted to the hospital with a 102-degree fever of unknown origin. According to standard procedure, his nurse, Jean, re-

121

moved the blankets from the bed, leaving only a sheet to cover him. She explained that it was to keep his temperature from going up. She gave him a glass of cold apple juice, but he only took two sips. At 9 P.M., the doctor examined Mr. Tomita and prescribed a mild analgesic every four hours for temperatures greater than 101 degrees and a cooling blanket for temperatures greater than 102 degrees. When his temperature rose to 103 degrees at 10 P.M., Jean ordered a cooling blanket, per the doctor's instructions. At this point, Mr. Tomita asked for his blankets, but Jean refused, once more explaining why. She put the ice blanket under him and left the room. In a few minutes, Mr. Tomita complained that the ice blanket was too cold and asked for his regular blankets. For the third time, Jean patiently explained the treatment. He did not say anything; he simply curled up under his sheet. When Jean returned a half hour later to check on him, he was sitting up in the chair with all the blankets wrapped around him, covered with goose bumps and shivering. By midnight, his temperature was up to 105 degrees. Jean gave him his second dosage of acetaminophen. Mr. Tomita continued to ask for his blankets and to get out of bed. Jean was at the point of putting restraints on him to keep him in bed.

She asked him why he did not want to stay in bed. He explained that in Japan, people with fevers were covered with warm blankets and given plenty of hot drinks. Cold juice was particularly inappropriate. This approach, found throughout Asia, is probably based on the Chinese notion of hot and cold balance, or yin and yang. Mr. Tomita was experiencing chills, which logically should be treated with heat, not cold. Furthermore, it is believed that fevers must be sweated out, again necessitating measures that produce greater warmth.

Reflecting on his comment, Jean asked herself what she did when suffering from a temperature and chills. She realized that she did exactly what her patient wanted—she piled lots of blankets on herself, turned up the electric blanket to the maximum temperature, and drank hot liquids!

She then called a team conference. Most of her colleagues admitted to similar behavior, but no one wanted to take responsibility for going against medical orders. Realizing that she could no longer treat Mr. Tomita against his beliefs and wishes, Jean decided to call the admitting doctor. It was now 1 A.M. The physician was angry at being awakened. He impatiently listened to her story, was silent for a moment, and then agreed to a change in orders: discontinue the cooling blanket, administer analgesic tablets every three hours if the patient's temperature rose above 101 degrees, and keep the patient as comfortable as possible.

Mr. Tomita was extremely happy and grateful for the change in orders. His temperature came down after about three hours and eventually he removed the blankets on his own.

A similar case involved Rosa Torres, a twenty-nine-year-old Hispanic woman with a surgical infection. Rosa's temperature was 104 degrees. She had piled six blankets on top of herself, curled up into a ball, and lay there moaning loudly. When Rebecca, her nurse, discovered the mound of blankets, she attempted to remove them. Rosa vehemently refused. "No, I will get cold." Rebecca explained that the blankets were keeping her body temperature too high; she needed to remove them to reduce the fever. The explanation did nothing to change Rosa's mind, but Rebecca was determined and gently pulled off all but one blanket.

Shortly thereafter, Rebecca tried to take Rosa's temperature rectally, per the doctor's orders. Again, Rosa refused. She did not want her underwear removed and certainly did not want anyone to insert a rectal thermometer. Each of Rebecca's attempts to do so were met with screams. Rebecca tried to explain the importance of the greater accuracy of the rectal temperature, but Rosa did not care. Rebecca finally gave up, respecting Rosa's right to refuse. Another nurse on the unit, however, was not about to give in to the patient's desires and insisted that she remove her underwear. She managed to insert the thermometer despite Rosa's cries and tears.

Although Rebecca did not understand the reason for Rosa's behavior at the time, she later learned from several Hispanic friends that it is believed that one of the greatest dangers during a fever is letting in cold air. Removing all the covers thus put the patient at risk. Second, the illness is seen as a kind of poison. Keeping the blankets on causes the body to sweat out the poison; thus, the fever goes down and the illness disappears. Rosa's refusal to remove her underwear and have her temperature taken rectally was probably due to the modesty typically found among Hispanic women.

Unlike the previous example, in which the nurse finally did respect the patient's wishes, in this case, Western medicine won out. Rosa was labeled a difficult patient because of her desire to adhere to her traditional beliefs regarding treatment of disease. Rebecca later suggested that the doctor could have been called to change the order from a rectal to an oral temperature. She still felt it was necessary to remove the blankets but thought that if she had understood Rosa's reasons, she might have been more empathetic.

In another case, a Mexican-American mother refused to use cooling measures in caring for her febrile infant, despite medical instructions to do so. Mrs. Lopez had called the hospital because her infant's temperature was very high. She was told to give the baby a mild analgesic and a cool bath and then to bring her in. Mrs. Lopez ignored both cooling instructions and, to the consternation of the medical staff, brought the child wrapped in several layers of blankets, outer garments, undershirt, and several pairs of socks. When asked why she did not follow the instructions given her, she replied, "He must sweat the fever out. Besides, he could get pneumonia from the night air and die."

Nurses who work in hospitals serving a large Hispanic population say that they see this behavior quite frequently. In fact, the sight of a family walking up to the registration window with a bundle of blankets in their arms usually prompts the nurses to prediagnose the child as having a fever and admit it right away. Immediate action is necessary to make sure the baby does not have a seizure while the family is registering.

Parents are generally willing to listen to the nurses' explanations on how to treat fevers in infants. The problem is often with their own parents. One young woman explained that she knew she should not wrap her baby so heavily, but her mother-in-law "made her do it." She had attended some parenting classes and knew the proper procedure but felt it was too difficult to fight the whole family. Health education is the only way to deal with such situations, but it will not be easy to overcome years of tradition.

124

Another example occurred with a Black woman and her tiny grandson. The child was brought into the hospital by his mother, Mary, and grandmother Adele Wilson. The nurse explained that she would put the naked infant in a cool mist tent and bathe him in cold water to reduce his temperature. Mary was quiet, calm, and cooperative. She indicated her concern by asking several questions about her son's condition.

Adele Wilson, however, did not appear to be listening. She got up from her chair, looked into the tent, and said, "You forgot to give him a blanket. That thing is real cold inside." The nurse again explained that she was keeping him cool because of his high temperature. Mary tried to calm her mother-in-law, seeing that she was becoming hostile. "Mama, it's okay." Mrs. Wilson responded, "What you talkin' 'bout? They got you believing in this foolishness too. I'm gonna put his blanket on him 'cause he is cold. I raised all my nine children and I never put one in no ice box. You know you need to wrap him so he can sweat the fever out. Hot chamomile tea would bring that fever down."

Most of the nurses dealt with the grandmother by avoiding her. They could not talk to her without arguing. How might they have handled the situation? They might have begun by asking her how she would have treated the child. They could have acknowledged her approach, which comes from years of use of natural remedies within the Black culture. They might also have incorporated her recommendation of chamomile tea. Mrs. Wilson's hostility may have been a reaction to what she perceived as racism on the part of the white nurses. A bit more respect on the part of the nurses might have helped.

Pica

Ruth Clay, a twenty-eight-year-old paraplegic Black female with two children craved Argo laundry starch while she was hospitalized following an auto accident. Since she had few visitors, she asked the staff to bring her the starch. The staff, who thought this craving was "crazy," told her they did not have any. Furthermore, her renal disease dictated a limited diet.

Ruth became very depressed during her long hospitalization. Finally, a young Black female physician was assigned to her case. Recognizing Ruth's craving as a cultural practice, she recommended that the grateful patient be allowed a small amount.

Eating laundry starch is a common form of pica—a craving for nonfood substances—among Black women, who often consume it during pregnancy. Some think it helps "build up the blood." Others say it keeps the baby's skin "clean." (It has a smooth, clean feel.) Still others believe it helps settle the stomach. (The consistency is reminiscent of chalky antacids.) This practice is a carryover from the slave tradition of eating dirt. The clay dirt in the South is rich in iron, and the craving is generally thought to be due to anemia or iron deficiency. (In truth, the ferric—Fe^3—form of iron [red, rust] is virtually unabsorbable and of no nutritional use. The absorbable form is the ferrous—Fe^4—ion. Therefore, eating soil would be of no nutritional value, even in iron deficiency anemia.) When Blacks moved out of the South, Argo starch (probably the major brand of laundry starch at the time) was substituted.

Although the circumstances under which the patient craved laundry starch were unusual, her choice of that particular nonfood item was not. In her mind, it may have been associated with a happier time—pregnancy—and thus brought her some consolation during this very difficult time. Psychologically, this is similar to the common practice of eating "comfort foods" when we are depressed. These are the special foods that our mothers made us eat when we were children, foods we associate with love and warmth.

Folk Healers

Another potential area for misunderstanding or confusion involves the use of folk healers. A sixty-year-old Black woman named Pearl Smith was admitted to the critical care unit with severe diarrhea and dehydration. All tests and exploratory surgery were negative. In desperation, the family called in a voodoo doctor. The staff reacted with disbelief, especially since the patient was educated and upper middle class. How could they seriously consult a "witch doctor"?

Since orthodox medicine had ruled out all medical causes, the only other possibility was a magical cause. Perhaps someone had put a hex on Mrs. Smith. Belief in voodoo often persists in Black culture, despite education and social class—just as do superstitious beliefs in Anglo culture. Like most ethnic groups, Blacks use multiple health care systems.

Did voodoo succeed where orthodox medicine failed? In this case, both systems were unsuccessful. Mrs. Smith continued to waste away and died several months after the onset of her illness.

127   The story of an eighty-three-year-old Cherokee Indian woman named Mary Cloud has a happier ending. Her grandson Joe brought her into the hospital emergency room after she had passed out at home. Lab tests and x-rays indicated that she had a bowel obstruction. After consulting with Joe, the attending physician called in a surgeon to remove it. Joe was willing to sign consent for the surgery, but it would not be legal; the patient had to sign for herself. Mrs. Cloud however, refused; she wanted to see the medicine man on the reservation. Unfortunately, it was an hour and a half drive each way, and she was too ill to be moved. Finally, the social worker suggested that the medicine man be brought to the hospital.

Joe left and drove to the reservation. About three hours later he returned, accompanied by a man in full traditional dress, complete with feather headdress, rattles, and bells. He entered Mrs. Cloud's room and for forty-five minutes conducted a healing ceremony. Outside the closed door, the stunned and amused staff could hear bells, rattles, chanting, and singing.

At the conclusion of the ceremony, the medicine man informed the doctor that Mrs. Cloud would now sign the consent form. She did and was immediately taken to surgery. Her recovery was uneventful and without complications.

What was responsible for her recovery? The hospital staff were sure it was the skill of the surgeon; Mrs. Cloud was convinced it was a result of the power of the medicine man. In any case, without the medicine man she would not have agreed to the surgery, or if she had, her attitude might have been so poor as to interfere with recovery. This is a perfect example of how traditional healers and physicians can successfully work together in the care of patients.

Proper Medical Treatment

Although not technically in the realm of folk medicine, an interesting   128
situation involved a forty-six-year-old Cambodian woman who came
into the hospital emergency room complaining of a growth in her
abdomen. After five days of testing, the staff finally discovered that
Mrs. Sok had not had a bowel movement in ten days. A laxative helped
some, but she was not happy with the care she was receiving and did
not feel she was getting better. When the physician became aware of
her enlarged spleen, he did a bone marrow biopsy. This extremely
painful procedure involves inserting a large needle into the bone and
aspirating tissue. When the biopsy was completed, Mrs. Sok thanked
the doctor profusely, saying she now felt much better.

What accounts for the sudden change in her attitude and percep-
tion of her health following this unpleasant procedure? In Cambodia,
injections are very common. Since Mrs. Sok had not received one, she
felt her care was inadequate and thus she would not get well. She
mistook the biopsy for a shot and concluded that she was now on the
road to recovery.

Proper Diagnosis

The American legal and medical systems recognize patients' right to
know all the details of their condition. The high incidence of medical
malpractice suits also dictates that physicians share all possible complications of any surgical procedure or medication. Such openness and
honesty can have a negative effect when dealing with patients from
other ethnic groups.

In China and Japan, where doctors are seen as authority figures in   129
a hierarchical and patriarchal society, patients are told little about their
condition. Lawsuits are extremely rare. The physician is expected to
know best and to use good judgment. If the patient has cancer, the
family might be told, but the patient is rarely given the diagnosis.
Asians have a tremendous fear of cancer, perceiving it as a death
sentence, even though many forms can be successfully treated. Patients
told they have cancer often mistakenly assume the situation is hopeless
and give up. Loss of will to live can lead to premature death.

Imagine the situation of a Chinese or Japanese patient new to the
United States, who is told he has cancer. The physician may believe it is
easily treatable through a combination of surgery, radiation, and chemotherapy. The patient, knowing that doctors never tell a patient he
has cancer, assumes the worst. He is going to die immediately. The
psychological ramifications can be devastating.

It would be best for the physician in such a case to talk with the family first about the success rate of the treatment to be undertaken. Perhaps a more technical term than "cancer," which would cover the physician's legal obligation but would not frighten the patient so much, could be used to describe his condition. In any case, anticipating the patient's response and proceeding with that in mind should do much to relieve the situation.

Body Image

Hair

130   A thirty-four-year-old Greek named Dimitri Sirkis was rushed to intensive care following a traffic accident. He was alert but obviously drunk. Alan, his nurse, explained that he would have to shave a few patches of chest hair so he could attach the electrocardiogram electrodes. Hospital policy required that all intensive care patients be put on a monitor. Mr. Sirkis became very agitated. He did *not* want his chest hair shaved. It took several explanations before Alan could persuade him to cooperate. He later explained his resistance. In Greece, a man's body hair is linked to his manhood. Mr. Sirkis had especially dark, thick hair, and shaving diminished his sense of virility.

Most of the nurses thought Mr. Sirkis was ridiculous and made sarcastic comments about his machismo. When Alan defended him, the laughter and comments were redirected toward him. Alan suggested that when male patients are reluctant to have their chest shaved, electrodes be placed on the back of their shoulders. Perhaps it took a male nurse to truly understand Mr. Sirkis's feelings.

131   A nurse named Susan had a much more dramatic encounter when she attempted to shave a seventy-two-year-old Sikh from India. The patient, Raj Singh, had been admitted after a heart attack. He was scheduled for a heart catheterization to determine the extent of the blockage in his coronary arteries. The procedure involved running a catheter up the femoral artery, located in the groin, and then passing it into his heart where special x-rays could be taken. His son was a cardiologist on staff and had explained the procedure to him in detail.

Susan entered Mr. Singh's room and explained that she had to shave his groin to prevent infection from the catheterization. As she pulled the razor from her pocket, she was suddenly confronted with the sight of shining metal flashing in front of her. Mr. Singh had a short sword in his hand and was waving it at her as he spoke excitedly in his native tongue. Susan got the message. She would *not* shave his groin.

She put away her "weapon," and he did the same. Susan, thinking the problem was that she was a woman, said she would get a male orderly to shave him. Mr. Singh's eyes lit up again as he angrily yelled, "No shaving of hair by anyone!"

Susan managed to calm him down by agreeing. She then called her supervisor and the attending physician to report the incident. The physician said he would do the procedure on an unshaved groin. At that moment, Mr. Singh's son stopped by. When he heard what had happened, he apologized profusely for not explaining his father's orthodox Sikh customs.

The Sikh religion forbids cutting or shaving any bodily hair. Orthodox Sikhs always carry a dagger with them, lest someone try to force them to do something against their religion—as Susan had. The dagger is considered one of the five "outer badges." The others are wearing hair and beard unshorn; wearing a turban; wearing knee-length pants; and wearing a steel bracelet on the right wrist. These badges reflect the Sikhs' military history.

Many of the procedures medical professionals consider necessary are not; when they conflict with patients' religious beliefs, they can be worked around. The doctor might have been willing to make compromises in Mr. Singh's case because his son was a member of the staff. All patients should be treated with the same respect.

A Native American woman named Estelle Begay brought her fifteen-month-old granddaughter Elena into the emergency room. The child was suffering from severe dehydration and fever. To restore fluids intravenously, the nurse shaved Elena's right temple and inserted an intravenous line. Mrs. Begay was busy filling out admitting papers while this was done. When she reached the unit to see her granddaughter, she became very anxious and upset. The nurse tried to reassure her that the intravenous lines were temporary and that as soon as the problem was corrected, the child would be fine. Mrs. Begay responded with sorrow and resignation. "She's going to die." The nurse tried to reassure her, but Mrs. Begay would not leave Elena's bedside.

At one point, Mrs. Begay did leave for a few hours. She returned with two relatives and a "medicine bundle," which she tried to put on Elena's bed. This was against hospital policy, however, and was not permitted. The nurse said she could leave it by the window, if she desired.

Mrs. Begay and the other relatives, who were no longer permitted in the unit except during limited visiting hours, kept a vigil outside the door. The next day, despite Elena's improvement, Mrs. Begay insisted upon taking her home against medical advice.

The following day, Elena was readmitted by her mother. She was still feverish and would not eat. A small bundle was attached to the child's shirt. As the nurse started to remove it, the mother stopped her.

132

"Please let her keep it. It is our custom." She went on to explain why Mrs. Begay had taken the child home against medical advice. She was afraid Elena would die.

"In our culture, it is taboo to cut a child's hair. Long, thick hair is a sign of a healthy child. To cut or shave it means the child will become sick or die." Mrs. Begay had gotten a medicine bundle to counteract the effect of violating the taboo but was not permitted to put it next to the child. It was useless sitting by the window. Mrs. Begay had no recourse but to take Elena home, where she could use the curative charm. This time, the nurses agreed to let the medicine bundle be placed next to Elena. After four days, her condition improved and she was able to go home.

This example illustrates two important points. Whenever a patient has something out of the ordinary, it probably has important religious significance and should not be removed. Second, many cultures have prohibitions against cutting hair, as was illustrated in the cases involving Mr. Sirkis and Mr. Singh. The biblical tale of Samson, who lost his strength when his hair was cut, reflects a similar taboo. In the 1960s, long hair on men symbolized their rebellion against mainstream American values. It is unclear why so much importance is attached to hair. It is interesting to note, however, that humans are the *only* primate species whose head hair grows constantly.

Scars

133   Most Americans are concerned with their appearance. Surgeons, therefore, try to leave as small a scar as possible. This effort had a negative effect with a forty-one-year-old Nigerian patient named Osito Seisay, who was introduced in Chapter 2. He had come to the United States to have his brother operate on his knee, which was injured when a bull charged him.

His nurse was concerned when he did not request pain medication following surgery. She learned the reason when his sister-in-law came to visit and spoke to Mr. Seisay in his native language. He was enduring the pain as an offering to Allah.

The next cultural incident occurred when Mr. Seisay's brother, the surgeon, came to remove the bandages. He was very proud of his work and pointed out how small the surgical scar was. Mr. Seisay, however, did not share his brother's happiness. He was disappointed over the small size of the scar. He felt that without a large scar to mark the surgery, the other members of his tribe would not believe he had suffered very much. What kind of offering to Allah would that be?

His brother had obviously shed most of the old tribal ways. He could not believe Osito still held these beliefs and tried in vain to convince him otherwise. At this point, nothing could be done. One would think that Mr. Seisay's brother, being aware of tribal customs, would have anticipated Osito's response. He did not. He was too Westernized. Surgeons, however, should be aware that all patients do not share the same ideal body image and should discuss such things in advance.

Fat

Mention of ideal body image brings up the subject of fat. American culture values thinness and views obesity as a disease. Many cultures, however, see thinness as a problem and plumpness as the ideal. Jane, a nurse, was about fifty pounds overweight. She was embarrassed about her size and eventually managed to lose most of the excess weight. She related an incident that occurred when she was at her heaviest.   134

Her Panamanian boyfriend, Mario, brought her home to meet his family. When they saw her, they were delighted that she was so fat. They told her this several times during the evening. Jane was totally humiliated by their remarks. She was already nervous about meeting Mario's family, and now they were insulting her. Yet they seemed so friendly.

Near the end of the evening, Mario, sensing her discomfort, took her aside and explained. In his culture, fat is seen as healthy. A fat woman can have lots of babies. All his other girlfriends had been far too thin to suit his family. At last, he was going out with a "real woman." They had not been insulting her by calling her fat; they were bestowing a great compliment. His explanation made Jane feel a little better, though their repeated comments about her size continued to disturb her.

Although this incident did not take place in the hospital, it illustrates a problem that could arise there. Most Latin Americans and Eastern Europeans, among others, share Mario's family's view of body size. Advice that a patient lose weight might not be followed because it would create a negative body image. Imagine a slim American woman being told she should gain twenty-five pounds for the sake of her health. How willing would she be to trade her "attractive" figure for one that she sees as too fat? Health care professionals should be aware of possible resistance and be prepared to deal with it.

Bathroom Behavior

The last incident to be discussed in this chapter does not fit neatly into any of the categories covered. It involves elimination. The patient,   135

Hyun Kim, a seventy-four-year-old Korean man, had come to the United States to visit his family. While here, he became ill and had to be hospitalized for renal and respiratory failure. He was put on strict bed rest because exertion would be dangerous. Conflict arose because several times a day, his family got him out of bed to squat over the bedpan on the floor. Kate, his nurse, tried to explain that the bedpan was to be used in bed, but they did not speak much English and became very upset. Kate was mystified over Mr. Kim's behavior.

A Filipino co-worker later explained. In most Asian countries, traditional toilets are holes in the ground. To eliminate from the bowels, one squats over the hole. There is no other way to do it. Until recently, most people did not have toilets inside their homes; they were located outside. Even today, the toilet is kept separate from the tub or shower. One is for cleansing, the other for waste. Elimination is considered unclean and certainly should not be done in bed. Mr. Kim's family was simply trying to maintain standards of cleanliness and decency. Mr. Kim was using the bedpan in the only way he knew how.

Once Kate understood his behavior, she drew the curtains around him for privacy. She then spoke to the physician and had him rewrite the orders from strict bedrest to bathroom privileges as needed with assistance. Mr. Kim and his family were much happier and more cooperative as a result. Kate also felt better because she was no longer frustrated over her lack of control.

More than once I have had the experience of going into a public restroom, checking the floor of the stalls for an empty one and, having found it, opened the door to find an Asian woman with her feet on the seat, squatting over the toilet. It is biomechanically easier to move the bowels in this position and is common in many parts of the world where Western plumbing is not found—and, occasionally, where it is. I was in a museum in southern France several years ago. I went to use the restroom but could not find the toilet. Finally, someone pointed out a hole in the ground. There were depressions on either side in the shape of footprints. I had to overcome a great deal of ethnocentrism before I was able to use it. The experience did, however, help me to be more understanding when I open a stall door to discover a woman with her feet on the toilet seat.

Summary

Most medical personnel believe that Western scientific medicine is superior to all other medical systems. In some cases, this may be true. It is important to remember, however, that medical practitioners in other cultures have been treating patients with some success for centuries.

Several modern drugs, including quinine, were discovered in native "medicine kits." Furthermore, scientific medicine has been notably unsuccessful in curing many ailments, including the common cold.

Even in cases where Western scientific medicine is superior, if the patient believes it is insufficient for treating the problem, it probably will be. The mind has a powerful effect on the body and can influence both illness and health. To treat patients successfully, it is extremely important to take their beliefs into account, whether they be about the causes of disease, how it should be treated, what behavior is appropriate, or how the body is viewed.

Ideally, medical professionals everywhere will recognize the value of what other systems have to offer. They can then take the best of each and reach the ultimate goal of providing effective health care for all.

Chapter 8
Conclusion

The examples in this book are by no means exhaustive. They represent a small sampling of the problems that can occur between members of different ethnic groups. Many of the basic principles that are illustrated by the examples can help in interpreting other conflicts or, ideally, preventing further misunderstandings. The works listed in the bibliography should help the interested reader research other aspects of cultural differences.

One of the issues that often arises in class discussions is that of ethics. Why should the Western health care system adapt to the needs of other cultural groups? We hear complaints such as, "Why don't they adapt to our ways?" "Why don't they learn to speak English? My grandparents did." Certainly, hospitals in most other countries are not nearly so accommodating to patients of other cultures.

One response is to say, yes, they *should* adapt to our culture and learn our language. That is not, however, the most compassionate or practical response. It is the goal of the medical profession to provide optimal health care for all patients. Unless cultural differences are taken into account, this goal cannot be accomplished. Misunderstandings can sometimes lead to misdiagnoses, as in the case of coin rubbing. Danger signals may be overlooked with a stoic Irish or Japanese patient.

The most important underlying message of this book is that cultural behavior is generally a result of adaptation to both the physical and the social environment. Different countries have different conditions—different weather, population size, vegetation, political circumstances, economic bases, and so forth. Cultures develop norms, values, and behaviors that are suited to these conditions. Over time, they take on the strength of tradition. Even when circumstances change, traditions often do not.

We are socialized by our culture at an early age. Early conditioning is very hard to overcome. Even when we move to a new country, where the customs and values are different, it is hard to change, even under the best of circumstances. Illness, particularly illness that requires hospitalization, is far from the best of circumstances. On the contrary, it is the very time when we are most likely to regress and behave in ways that were reinforced in childhood.

Certainly it is best for people to speak the language of the country in which they are living. Unfortunately, many immigrants to this country work long hours every day at physical labor. They are often too tired at night to attend English classes. Furthermore, they tend to live in ethnic communities where everyone speaks their native language, and thus they have no pressing need to learn English. Finally, not everyone has an equal facility with language. English is difficult to learn. The rules are far more irregular than in the Romance languages such as Spanish. It is much easier for children to learn new languages, perhaps because they are not so inhibited or afraid to make mistakes as adults are. For many people, the idea of learning a difficult new language may be overwhelming. So though ideally everyone in the United States should speak English, many do not. Does that mean they should receive inferior care?

Whether patients should speak English and adapt to our ways is irrelevant. The fact is that they do not and may not. The options are to provide inferior medical care (and experience high levels of stress resulting from frustration) or to make accommodations so as to provide optimal care (while at the same time reducing stress and frustration).

The anecdotes in this book were chosen to illustrate some of the most common or difficult problems that occur in hospitals as a result of cultural differences. In some instances, knowledge can prevent problems from occurring, as in the case of dietary taboos or preferences. In other cases, merely understanding *why* patients act the way they do may help hospital personnel be more compassionate and experience less frustration. Although at times it may appear that a patient's sole goal is to make things difficult for nurses and doctors, this is rarely the case. The patients are merely behaving in ways they were taught were appropriate or that were successful at other times in their lives.

In summary I will highlight the important points of the six preceding chapters.

Communication and Time Orientation

When choosing an interpreter, it is not enough for the person to speak the same language as the patient. It is important to choose someone of the appropriate sex and relationship. Same-sex interpreters are usually best.

Eye contact may have different meaning in different cultures. Lack of eye contact may reflect respect or concern rather than disinterest.

Idioms should be avoided whenever possible. Also remember that all English is not the same. The same words may have different meanings in different English-speaking countries, for example "fanny" and "fag" (the latter is a cigarette in England). The identity of the speaker is also important. A Black person may refer to a Black man as a "boy," but it would be very inappropriate for a Caucasian to do so.

A patient should be referred to as Mr., Mrs., Miss, or Ms. unless told by the patient to do otherwise. People suffer tremendous loss of dignity when they become patients; it is important not to add unnecessarily to this loss.

Remember that "yes" may not always mean the affirmative; for an Asian, it may be a way of avoiding the embarrassment of saying "no." Or, it may be the grammatically correct but misleading answer to a negative question, as in, "Haven't you eaten yet today?" It is best to ask open-ended questions and to avoid negatives whenever possible. Also be aware that masculine and feminine pronouns do not exist in many Asian languages, and interpret statements accordingly.

Try not to use gestures, because many of those with neutral or even positive connotations in the United States ("okay," "thumbs up," and "victory") may have insulting or sexually suggestive connotations elsewhere.

Some cultures encourage emotional expressiveness while others encourage emotional control. Ascertain whether the individual is a typical representative of his or her culture and, if so, adjust the attention given accordingly. It may be necessary to anticipate the pain needs of an Asian or Irish patient and not become overly concerned with the moans of a Mediterranean or Middle Eastern patient.

People from many cultures may be reluctant to discuss anything about their personal life or problems. Hispanic patients may feel it is the business only of other family members, not strangers. Asian patients may be trying to avoid the stigma of mental illness. Gypsy patients may simply not trust outsiders.

Time orientation varies among different ethnic groups (as well as among individuals). Present-oriented individuals may be late for appointments. Tardiness may be compounded by poverty; reliance on public transportation and difficulties in getting time off from work may also contribute to this problem. In addition, people with a present time orientation may not practice preventive health care, and those with a past orientation may be reluctant to try new techniques.

Religion and Beliefs

Religion is often an integral part of people's lives, becoming even more important during times of illness. Patients' religious beliefs should be respected and incorporated into their care whenever possible. Time should be set aside for the patient to pray undisturbed, if so desired.

Some religions have beliefs that conflict with Western medicine, for example, Jehovah's Witnesses' beliefs about blood transfusions. When confronted with such conflicts, consider the patients' perspective and the possibility that their beliefs may be correct. Also remember that they live within a social network. The social cost of violating religious taboos may be too high for them to be willing to do so.

Hospital staff may also have religious beliefs that interfere with some medical practices, as in the case of a Catholic nurse who refused to assist in an abortion. Staff members should make such restrictions known to their supervisors, who in turn should respect them.

It is also important to be aware of holy days and restrictions associated with them, such as the Orthodox Jewish prohibition against any form of work on the Sabbath (Saturday).

Recognize that religious symbols can take many forms, from Catholic rosary beads to Mormon long underwear. These should not be removed without discussion, and it is best to try to keep them in contact with the patient's body whenever possible. This can be important psychologically to the patient.

Many religions and cultures have dietary taboos or prescriptions which should be ascertained at the intake interview. Muslims and Orthodox Jews are forbidden pork, Asians and Hispanics may be concerned about hot/cold body balance, and Filipinos may desire rice with every meal. It should not be assumed that a patient who refuses to eat lacks an appetite; it may just be that inappropriate foods were served. Suggest alternative foods to the patient or family.

People may hold beliefs regarding witchcraft or magic. Rather than ignore their beliefs, it is usually most effective to use them. Deal with patients within the context of their belief system, rather than outside it.

Numbers may have lucky or unlucky associations, which should be taken into account when assigning rooms. Japanese avoid the number 4; Navahos prefer it. Astrology may be important for some Asian patients, and it may play a role in determining when to remove life support.

Finally, expect Gypsies to light candles around the bed of a dying patient. Take precautions with regard to oxygen equipment.

Family

Most non-Anglo cultures value family highly. Many patients come from large families—a necessity in agricultural communities. When a family member is ill, the rest feel they must be there with the patient. For the well-being of the patient and the family, it is best to be as flexible as possible regarding visitors and visiting hours, setting limits when necessary. If possible, place patients with frequent large groups of visitors (such as Gypsies) in a room at the end of the hall, or where there will be minimum disturbance to other patients.

Self-care, a medical goal for patients, is often ignored. The family will often take over feeding and grooming the patient. This may be an important way for family members to demonstrate their love and respect for the patient. It may also be a way for a male patient from a hierarchical culture to demonstrate continued control over his family, despite physical weakness. If self-care is necessary for recovery—as in the case of burn patients—give the family tasks that will not impede the patient's progress. If the staff's emphasis on self-care is primarily a reflection of the American value of independence, do not insist but allow the family to continue caring for the patient.

Be sensitive to feelings of perceived racism among minority group members. As a result of years of slavery and discrimination, Blacks may be sensitive even to unintentional threats to their self-esteem.

Recognize that although it may be against hospital policy, many patients will try to give gifts to nurses, either to remove the debt of obligation or to ensure good service. It is best to accept such gifts but to encourage only those that can be shared by the entire nursing staff.

Realize that kinship systems may differ from that found among Anglo-Americans and that other relatives may be closer to a child than the biological parents. Hospital rules regarding who may sign informed consent will still have to be followed, but consult with appropriate relatives, such as grandparents or uncles, for example, in the case of a Navaho.

Men and Women

Few cultures share an egalitarian ideal for men and women. In most cultures, men are thought to be the heads of the house and the primary decision makers. This situation is gradually changing as a result of the spread of Western influence, but change is slow and sporadic.

Males may therefore serve as spokespersons for their wives; sons may dictate to their mothers. Male employees may refuse to take orders from a female supervisor. This behavior may have to be tolerated in patients; among staff, termination is an option if change does not follow open discussion of the problem.

In hierarchical cultures, age generally carries authority. Elders may make decisions for their grown children. Often it may be the best policy for hospital personnel to address their first remarks to the eldest family member present, rather than to the patient.

Culture may dictate appropriate behavior for each sex. For example, in Asian cultures, women are expected to be passive rather than assertive and to show respect for authority rather than challenge it. This can lead to problems in the hospital if an Asian woman is in a leadership position which requires assertiveness, especially when dealing with superiors. (If her basic nature is assertive, however, she may quickly overcome her early socialization.)

Some cultures, such as Asian or Middle Eastern, may prefer male children over females because males traditionally take care of parents when they are old, and they carry on the family name. The latter is especially important in cultures like Chinese that practice ancestor worship. Although hospital staff may be disturbed at seeing parents show preference for male children, they should not expect people to change.

Female purity is especially important in the Middle East and in Muslim countries in general. Intimate contact between the sexes is forbidden outside of marriage. The use of same-sex doctors and nurses will get the best results. Modesty is also a major concern in Hispanic, Asian, and Gypsy cultures; in fact, it is important in most cultures and should be respected. Although it is often not expedient to take the time to ensure a patient's personal privacy, it is a goal to strive for with all patients.

Birth

Though birth is a universal event, behavior during labor is strongly culturally conditioned. Women are taught to be loud or stoic, to push or not push during different times. Generally, cultures that value emotional expressiveness allow or encourage expressiveness during labor; those that value emotional control encourage stoicism during labor. Labor is not a time to try to change patients' behavior. If possible, women with similar levels of expressiveness should be put in the same room.

Labor attendants also vary cross-culturally. One should not assume that a woman's husband is the desired labor partner. In many cultures, including Asian and Hispanic, the woman's mother may be more appropriate. This matter can easily be discussed with the patient.

Many cultures practice a postpartum lying-in period during which time bathing and exercise are prohibited. Certain foods must be avoided while others are encouraged. Though with current Diagnostic Related Groups new mothers are rarely in the hospital long enough for this to be an issue, it should be taken into account, particularly with Asian, East Indian, and Hispanic women. Also try to avoid offering ice water, unless it is requested, because it may be thought to be too cold for a body that has just been depleted of heat through the process of giving birth. Be aware that young mothers may be willing to comply with Western medical recommendations but hesitate to do so in the presence of their more traditional mothers.

Bonding between mother and child is often a concern. Some cultures, such as Vietnamese, may appear to have bonding problems because of beliefs that spirits want to steal newborns. An apparent lack of attention may actually be an effort to thwart the interest of spirits. Health care professionals should follow the lead of the parents in their own displays of attention to infants. Apparent neglect may also be a part of the lying-in period. Among East Indians, for example, family members take over the care of the infant to allow the new mother time to recuperate.

Women from various cultures may wait several days before breast-feeding their newborns so as to allow their milk to come in. Since the early colostrum is important to the infant's health, patient education may be necessary to encourage early breastfeeding.

Birth control is often a sensitive issue because of religious prohibitions or simply its sexual nature. Some methods may be more accept-able than others, given concerns over modesty. It is important to give explicit instructions regarding how to use various methods; do not assume the patient will know what to do. Realize that husbands and wives may have different desires regarding family size and be sensitive to this in discussions of birth control and sterilization.

Folk Medicine

All cultures have developed their own methods for treating illness based on observed cause-and-effect relationships. Some techniques, such as coin rubbing and cupping, produce marks that may appear to be signs of child abuse or unrelated symptoms. It is important to recognize these before jumping to unwarranted conclusions.

Conventional wisdom generally treats fever by trying to sweat it out; Western medicine tries to cool it down. Patients may be very resistant to cooling measures. When such measures are used, the rationale for them should be carefully explained. First, however, consider the possibility that allowing the patient to have additional blankets may have an important psychological effect.

Patients may occasionally experience pica—a craving for non-food substances. A common pica among pregnant Black women is Argo laundry starch. The quantity consumed should be monitored for health reasons, but the psychological benefits of allowing a small amount may be substantial.

When doctors are unable to cure a patient or to obtain consent to certain procedures, it may be beneficial to honor a patient's request to bring in a traditional healer. Such healers are occasionally successful, whether from the efficaciousness of their treatments or a placebo effect.

Patients may hold beliefs regarding the effectiveness of certain medical procedures. Asians, for example, often feel that an injection is necessary for proper treatment. It might be helpful to ask patients' opinions regarding the treatment they feel will make them better. Hospital staff should realize that in cultures such as Asian or Native American, physicians are important authority figures. They should not have to ask the patient too many questions; a good doctor will know the answers. In such cases, it might be best for the nurse to ask questions of the patient.

Not all cultures share our open approach with patients, in part because of the authority of the physician and in part because malpractice suits are uncommon. Because many Asians have an almost irrational fear of cancer, it may be best to discuss such a diagnosis with the family before telling the patient.

Body image varies cross-culturally. "Beauty is in the eye of the beholder" is an old cliché but an accurate one nonetheless. Members of some cultures may value features Americans dislike, for example, scars or body fat. Do not assume that everyone shares our ideals. Fat may be seen as a sign of health and fertility in a culture where starvation and malnutrition are common.

Hair has significance in many cultures. It should not be shaved or cut without first discussing it with the patient. If the patient objects, alternatives should be sought.

Finally, remember that all toilets are not alike and that bathroom habits may vary. People from Third World and even some European countries may be used to squatting over a hole and may have difficulty using a toilet seat.

Summary

Transcultural health care requires a holistic and culturally relativistic approach. Treat the patient as a whole person with psychological and spiritual needs as well as physical ones. See patients as members of a family unit, not as just individuals. Do not assume that patients or co-workers will view the world the same way that you do; they may have different values and different ways of looking at things. Do not make assumptions and do respect differences. Recognize that other people's views are just as valid as yours.

If this advice were applied to all patients, no matter what their ethnic or cultural background, we would go a long way toward providing better care for patients from all cultures.

Selected Bibliography

General

Bauwens, E., ed. (1978) *The Anthropology of Health.* St. Louis: C. V. Mosby.

Berlin, E. A., and W. C. Fowkes, Jr. (1983) A teaching framework for cross-cultural health care: Application in family practice. *Western Journal of Medicine* 139: 928–933.

Boyle, J. S., and M. M. Andrews. (1989) *Transcultural Concepts in Nursing Care.* Boston: Scott, Foresman.

Branch, M. F., and P. P. Paxton. (1976) *Providing Safe Nursing Care for Ethnic People of Color.* New York: Appleton-Century-Crofts.

Brink, P. J. (1976) *Transcultural Nursing: A Book of Readings.* Englewood Cliffs, NJ: Prentice-Hall.

Brownlee, A. T. (1978) *Community, Culture and Care: A Cross Cultural Guide for Healthworkers.* St. Louis: C. V. Mosby.

Bullough, B., and V. L. Bullough. (1972) *Poverty, Ethnic Identity and Health Care.* New York: Appleton-Century-Crofts.

Bullough, V. L., and B. Bullough. (1982) *Health Care for Other Americans.* New York: Appleton-Century-Crofts.

Clark, M. M. (1983) Cultural context of medical practice. *Western Journal of Medicine* 139(6): 806–810.

Elling, R. H. (1977) *Socio-Cultural Influences on Health and Health Care.* New York: Springer.

Elliott, J. L. (1972) Cultural barriers to the utilization of health services. *Inquiry* 9: 28–35.

Foster, G. M., and B. G. Anderson. (1978) *Medical Anthropology.* New York: John Wiley & Sons.

Gorrie, M. (1989) Reaching clients through cross cultural education. *Journal of Gerontological Nursing* 15(10): 29–31.

Hartog, J., and E. A. Hartog. (1983) Cultural aspects of health and illness behavior in hospitals. *Western Journal of Medicine* 139: 910–916.

Harwood, A. (1981) *Ethnicity and Medical Care.* Cambridge: Harvard University Press.

Henderson, G., and M. Primeaux, eds. (1981) *Transcultural Health Care.* Menlo Park, CA: Addison-Wesley.

Kim, S. S. (1983) Ethnic elders and American health care: A physician's perspective. *Western Journal of Medicine* 139: 885–891.

Klein, N., ed. (1979) *Culture, Curers & Contagion.* Novato, CA: Chandler & Sharp.

Kleinman, A., L. Eisenberg, and B. Good. (1978) Culture, illness and care: Clinical lessons. Anthropologic and cross-cultural research. *Annals of Internal Medicine* 88: 251–258.

Leininger, M. (1970) *Nursing and Anthropology: Two Worlds to Blend.* New York: John Wiley.

Leininger, M. (1978) *Transcultural Nursing: Concepts, Theories and Practices.* New York: John Wiley.

Mindel, C. H., and R. W. Habenstein, eds. (1976) *Ethnic Families in America.* New York: Elsevier.

Moore, L., P. Van Arsdale, J. Glittenberg, and R. Aldrich. (1980) *The Biocultural Basis of Health.* St. Louis: C. V. Mosby.

Orque, M. S., B. Bloch, and L. S. A. Monrroy. (1983) *Ethnic Nursing Care: A Multicultural Approach.* St. Louis: C. V. Mosby.

Payer, L. (1988) *Medicine and Culture.* New York: Henry Holt.

Rackovsky, I. (1980, July) Nurses, nursing and culture. *Supervisor Nurse,* pp. 20–22.

Read, M. (1966) *Culture, Health and Disease.* London: Tavistock.

Ruiz, M. C. J. (1981) Open-closed mindedness, intolerance of ambiguity and nursing faculty attitudes toward culturally different patients. *Nursing Research* 30(3): 177–181.

Saunders, L. (1954) *Cultural Differences and Medical Care.* New York: Sage.

Smith, S. (1989) People without land. *American Journal of Nursing* 89(2): 208–209.

Spector, R. E. (1985) *Cultural Diversity in Health and Illness.* Norwalk, CT: Appleton-Century-Crofts.

Spicer, E. H., ed. (1977) *Ethnic Medicine in the Southwest.* Tucson: University of Arizona Press.

Valente, S. M. (1989, September) Overcoming cultural barriers. *California Nurse,* pp. 4–5.

Journals

Journal of Transcultural Nursing
Medical Anthropology Quarterly
Medical Anthropology

Ethnic Groups

ASIANS AND EAST INDIANS

Abu-Saad, H., J. Kayser-Jones, and J. Tien. (1982) Asian nursing students in the United States. *Journal of Nursing Education* 21(7): 11–15.

Anderson, J. N. (1983) Health and illness in Pilipino immigrants. *Western Journal of Medicine* 139: 811–819.

Bowers, J. Z. (1965) *Medical Education in Japan.* New York: Harper & Row.

Campbell, T., and B. Chang. (1981) Health care of the Chinese in America. In G. Henderson and M. Primeaux, eds., *Transcultural Health Care*, pp. 162–171. Menlo Park, CA: Addison-Wesley.

Chang, B. (1981) Asian-American patient care. In G. Henderson and M. Primeaux, eds., *Transcultural Health Care*, pp. 255–278. Menlo Park, CA: Addison-Wesley.

Chen-Louie, T. (1983) Nursing care of Chinese American patients. In M. S. Orque, B. Bloch, and L. S. A. Monrroy, eds., *Ethnic Nursing Care: A Multicultural Approach*, pp. 183–218. St. Louis: C. V. Mosby.

Clayton, J., and A. Henley. (1982, August) Asians in the hospital: Illness and the life cycle. *Health and Social Services Journal*, pp. 972–974.

De Gracia, R. (1979, December) Health care of the American Asian patient. *Critical Care Update*, p. 19.

Dyck, B. (1989) The paper crane. *American Journal of Nursing* 89(6): 824–825.

Ellis, J. (1982) Southeast Asian refugees and maternity care: The Oakland experience. *Birth* 9(3): 191–194.

Gonzales, N. (1966) Filipino culture and food habits. *Philippine Journal of Nutrition* 19: 194–201.

Gordon, V. D., I. M. Matousek, and T. A. Lang. (1980) Southeast Asian refugees: Life in America. *American Journal of Nursing* 80: 2031–2036.

Grippin, J. T. (1979) The Japanese American client. *Issues in Mental Health Nursing* 2: 57–69.

Hashizume, S., and J. Takano. (1983) Nursing care of Japanese American patients. In M. S. Orque, B. Bloch, and L. S. A. Monrroy, eds., *Ethnic Nursing Care*, pp. 219–243. St. Louis: C. V. Mosby.

Henderson, L. (1967) *Vietnam and Countries of the Mekong.* Camden, NJ: Thomas Nelson and Sons.

Hollingsworth, A., P. L. Brown, and D. A. Brooten. (1980) The refugees and childbearing: What to expect. *RN Magazine* 43: 45–48.

Kiefer, C. W. (1974) *Changing Cultures, Changing Lives: An Ethnographic Study of Three Generations of Japanese Americans.* San Francisco: Jossey-Bass.

Kitano, H. (1969) *Japanese-Americans.* Englewood Cliffs, NJ: Prentice-Hall.

Kleinman, A., P. Kunstader, E. R. Alexander, and J. Gale, eds., (1975) *Medicine in Chinese Cultures.* Washington, DC: Fogarty International Center

Kuhni, C. Q. (1990, January) When cultures clash at the bedside. *RN*, 23–26.

Landry, L. (1968) *The Land and People of Southeast Asia.* New York: J. B. Lippincott.

LeBar, F. and A. Suddard. (1960) *Laos: Its People, Its Society, Its Culture.* New Haven, CT: HRAF Press.

Lebra, T. S., and W. P. Lebra. (1974) *Japanese Culture and Behavior.* Honolulu: University of Hawaii Press.

Lee, R. (1970) *Chinese in America.* Hong Kong: Hong Kong University Press.

Leslie, C., ed. (1976) *Asian Medical Systems.* Los Angeles: University of California Press.

Leyn, R. B. (1978) The challenge of caring for child refugees from Southeast Asia. *American Journal of Maternal Child Nursing*, 3, 178–182.

Liu, W. T., M. Lamanna, and A. Muralta. (1979) *Transition to Nowhere: Vietnamese Refugees in America.* Nashville, TN: Charter House.

Lock, M. (1983) Japanese responses to social change: Making the strange familiar. *Western Journal of Medicine* 139: 829–834.

Longo, B. (1990, February 5) Confusing blend of Asian, U.S. medicine. *Nurse-week*, pp. 1, 22.

Muecke, M. A. (1983) In search of healers: Southeast Asian refugees in the American health care system. *Western Journal of Medicine* 129: 835–840.

Ohnuki-Tierney, E. (1984) *Illness and Culture in Contemporary Japan.* New York: Cambridge University Press.

Orque, M. S. (1983) Nursing care of Filipino American patients. In M. S. Orque, B. Bloch, and L. S. A. Monrroy, eds., *Ethnic Nursing Care: A Multicultural Approach,* pp. 149–181. St. Louis: C. V. Mosby.

Orque, M. S. (1983) Nursing care of South Vietnamese patients. In M. S. Orque, B. Bloch, and L. S. A. Monrroy, eds., *Ethnic Nursing Care: A Multicultural Approach,* pp. 245–270. St. Louis: C. V. Mosby.

Osgood, C. (1954) *The Koreans and Their Culture.* Tokyo: Houghton Mifflin.

Schacht, R. (1989) Epilogue: Glimpses of China and Chinese elders. *Journal of Gerontological Nursing* 15(1): 39–40.

Sheppard, H. (1990, February 5) How Hispanic cultural patterns affect care-givers. *Nurseweek,* pp. 15–16.

Tsung-Yi, L. (1983) Psychiatry and Chinese culture. *Western Journal of Medicine* 139: 862–867.

Wilson, D. K. (1980, November) The Refugee. *RN Magazine,* pp. 42–48.

Wolf, M. (1968) *Women in Chinese Society.* New York: Appleton-Century-Crofts.

BLACKS

Billingsley, A. (1968) *Black Families in White America.* Englewood Cliffs, NJ: Prentice-Hall.

Billingsley, A. (1974) *Black Families and the Struggle for Survival.* New York: Friendship Press.

Burgess, H. A. (1987) Into the Sudan. *American Journal of Nursing* 87(7): 927–929.

Harrison, I. E., and D. S. Harrison. (1971) The Black family experience and health behavior. In C. Crawford, ed., *Health and the Family.* New York: Macmillan.

Jones, E. L. (1976) Nursing care of the Black patient. In D. Luckraft, ed., *Black Awareness: Implications for Black Patient Care,* pp. 36–37. New York: American Journal of Nursing.

Lewis, D. K. (1975) The black family socialization and sex roles. *Phylon* 36: 221–237.

Luckraft, D., ed. (1976) *Black Awareness: Implications for Black Patient Care.* New York: American Journal of Nursing.

Martin, E. P., and J. M. Martin. (1978) *The Black Extended Family.* Chicago: University of Chicago Press.

Mays, R. M. (1979) Primary health care and the Black family. *Nurse Practitioner* 4: 13.

Meindl, N., and C. Getty. (1981) Life-styles of Black families headed by women. In C. Getty and W. Humphreys, eds., *Understanding the Family,* pp. 157–184. New York: Appleton-Century-Crofts.

Nobles, W. W., and G. M. Nobles. (1976) African roots in Black families: The social-psychological dynamics of Black family life and the implications for nursing care. In D. Luckraft, ed., *Black Awareness: Implications for Black Patient Care*, p. 19. New York: American Journal of Nursing.

Parker, S., and R. J. Kleiner, eds. (1966) *Mental Illness in the Urban Negro Community.* New York: Free Press.

Parsons, T., and K. B. Clark. (1965) *The American Negro.* Boston: Beacon Press.

Seham, M. (1973) *Blacks and American Medical Care.* Minneapolis: University of Minnesota Press.

Snow, L. F. (1977) Popular medicine in a Black neighborhood. In E. H. Spicer, ed., *Ethnic Medicine in the Southwest*, pp. 19–95. Tucson: University of Arizona Press.

Snow, L. F. (1983) Traditional health beliefs and practices among lower class Black Americans. *Western Journal of Medicine* 139: 820–828.

Thomas, D. N. (1981) Black American patient care. In G. Henderson and M. Primeaux, eds., *Transcultural Health Care.* Menlo Park, CA: Addison-Wesley.

Ullendorf, E. (1960) *The Ethiopians.* London: Oxford University Press.

White, E. (1974) Health and the Black person: An annotated bibliography. *American Journal of Nursing* 74: 1839–1841.

Williams, R. A. (1975) *Textbook of Black Related Diseases.* New York: McGraw-Hill.

GYPSIES

Anderson, G., and B. Tighe. (1979) Gypsy culture and health care. In N. Klein, ed., *Culture, Curers & Contagion*, pp. 195–200. Novato, CA: Chandler & Sharp.

Brink, S. (1988) Doctoring Gypsies. *Boston Magazine* 7: 80–86.

Clark, M. W. (1967) Vanishing vagabonds: The American Gypsies. *Texas Quarterly* 10: 204–210.

Clebert, J. P. (1969) *The Gypsies.* Baltimore: Penguin.

Cohn, W. (1973) *The Gypsies.* Reading, MA: Addison-Wesley.

Gropper, R. C. (1975) *Gypsies in the City.* Princeton, NJ: Darwin Press.

Kephart, W. M. (1989) The Gypsies. In E. Angeloni, ed., *Annual Editions: Anthropology 89/90*, pp. 122–137. Guilford, CT: Dushkin.

Manneli, F. (1974) Gypsies, culture and child care. *Pediatrics* 54(5): 603–607.

Sutherland, A. (1975) *Gypsies: The Hidden Americans.* New York: Free Press.

Sway, M. (1988) *Familiar Strangers: Gypsy Life in America.* Champaign: University of Illinois Press.

Webb, G. E. C. (1960) *Gypsies: The Secret People.* London: Herbert Jenkins.

Yoors, J. (1967) *Gypsies.* New York: Simon and Schuster.

HISPANICS

Baca, J. E. (1978) Some health beliefs of the Spanish speaking. In R. A. Martinez, ed., *Hispanic Culture and Health Care*, pp. 92–98. St. Louis: C. V. Mosby.

Barnett, S. E. (1980) Migrant health revisited: A model for statewide health planning and services. *American Journal of Public Health* 70: 1092–1094.

Burma, J. H., ed. (1970) *Mexican Americans in the United States.* Cambridge, MA: Schenkman.

Clark, M. (1959) *Health in the Mexican-American Culture.* Los Angeles: University of California Press.

Delgado, M., and D. Humm-Delgado. (1982) Natural support systems: Source of strength in Hispanic communities. *Social Work* 27: 83–89.

Diaz-Guerrero, R. (1955) Neurosis and the Mexican family structure. *American Journal of Psychiatry* 112: 411–417.

Grebler, L., J. W. Moore, and R. G. Guzman. (1970) *The Mexican-American People: The Nation's Second Largest Minority.* New York: Free Press.

Kay, M. A. (1977) Health and illness in a Mexican American barrio. In E. H. Spicer, ed., *Ethnic Medicine in the Southwest.* Tucson: University of Arizona Press.

Keefe, S., A. Padilla, and M. Carlos. (1979) The Mexican-American family as an emotional support system. *Human Organization* 38: 144–152.

Madsen, W. (1964) *The Mexican-Americans of South Texas.* New York: Holt, Rinehart & Winston.

Martinez, R. A. (1978) *Hispanic Culture and Health Care.* St. Louis: C. V. Mosby.

Mindel, C. (1980) Extended familism among urban Mexican Americans, Anglos and Blacks. *Hispanic Journal of Behavioral Sciences* 2: 21–34.

Monrroy, L. (1983) Nursing care of Raza/Latina patients. In M. S. Orque, B. Bloch, and L. Monrroy, eds., *Ethnic Nursing Care: A Multicultural Approach,* pp. 115–148. St. Louis: C. V. Mosby.

Murillo, N. (1978) The Mexican American Family. In R. A. Martinez, ed., *Hispanic Culture and Health Care,* pp. 3–18. St. Louis: C. V. Mosby.

Murillo-Rohde, I. (1981) Hispanic American patient care. In G. Henderson and M. Primeaux, eds., *Transcultural Health Care,* pp. 224–237. Menlo Park, CA: Addison-Wesley.

Nall, F. C., and J. Speilberg. (1967) Social and cultural factors in the responses of Mexican-Americans to medical treatment. *Journal of Health and Social Behavior* 8: 299–308.

Ramirez, S., and R. Parres. (1957) Some dynamic patterns in the organization of the Mexican family. *International Journal of Social Psychiatry* 3: 18–21.

Rubel, A. (1960) Concepts of disease in Mexican-American culture. *American Anthropologist* 62: 795–814.

Samora, J. (1978) Conception of health and disease among Spanish Americans. In R. Martinez, ed., *Hispanic Culture and Health Care,* pp. 65–74. St. Louis: C. V. Mosby.

Saunders, L. (1954) *Cultural Differences and Medical Care: The Case of the Spanish-Speaking People of the Southwest.* New York: Russell Sage Foundation.

Sharff, J. W. (1981) Free enterprise and the ghetto family. In E. Angeloni, ed., *Annual Editions: Anthropology 89/90,* pp. 117–121. Guilford, CT: Dushkin.

Steiner, S. (1969) *La Raza: The Mexican Americans.* New York: Harper & Row.

Teichner, V. J., J. J. Cadden, and G. W. Berry. (1981) The Puerto Rican patient: Some historical, cultural and psychosocial aspects. *Journal of the American Academy of Psychoanalysis* 9: 177–189.

Wagley, C. (1968) *The Latin American Tradition.* New York: Columbia University Press.

MIDDLE EASTERNERS

Berger, M. (1962) *The Arab World Today.* Garden City, NY: Doubleday.

Collins, R. O., and R. L. Tignor. (1967) *Egypt and the Sudan*. Englewood Cliffs, NJ: Prentice-Hall.

Eickelman, D. F. (1981) *The Middle East: An Anthropological Approach*. Englewood Cliffs, NJ: Prentice-Hall.

Fernea, E. W. and R. A. Fernea. (1989) A look behind the veil. In E. Angeloni, ed., *Annual Editions: Anthropology 89/90*, pp. 149–153. Guilford, CT: Dushkin.

Fitzsimmons, T., ed., (1959) *Saudi Arabia: Its People, Its Society, Its Culture*. New Haven, CT: HRAF Press.

Gibb, H. A. R. (1962) *Mohammedanism*. 2d ed. New York: Oxford University Press.

Goldschmidt, A. (1979) *A Concise History of the Middle East*. Boulder, CO: Praeger.

Good, B. J. (1977) The heart of what's the matter: The semantics of illness in Iran. *Culture, Medicine, & Psychiatry* 1: 25–28.

Haim, S. G., and Kedouri, E. (1980) *Towards a Modern Iran: Studies in Thought, Politics and Society*. London: Frank Cass.

Julali, B. (1982) Iranian families. In M. McGoldrick, ed., *Ethnicity and Family Therapy*, pp. 289–302. New York: Guilford Press.

Lipson, J. G., and A. I. Meleis. (1983) Issues in health care of Middle Eastern patients. *Western Journal of Medicine* 139: 854–861.

Mansfield, P., ed., (1980) *The Middle East*. 3d ed. New York: Oxford University Press.

Meleis, A. (1981) The Arab American in the health care system. *American Journal of Nursing* 81(6): 1180–1183.

Mills, A. C. (1986) Saudi Arabia: An overview of nursing and health care. *Focus on Critical Care* 13(1): 50–56.

Nicholls, P. H. (1989) Transplanted to Saudi Arabia. *American Journal of Nursing* 89(8): 1048–1050.

Patai, R. (1959) *Sex and Family in the Bible and the Middle East*. New York: Doubleday.

Patai, R. (1969) *Society, Culture and Change in the Middle East*. 3d ed. New York: Flecker.

Patai, R. (1973) *The Arab Mind*. New York: Scribner's.

Shiloh, A. (1968) The interaction between the Middle Eastern and Western systems of medicine. *Social Science Medicine* 2: 235–248.

Simpson-Hebert, M. (1989) Women, food and hospitality in Iranian society. In E. Angeloni, ed., *Annual Editions: Anthropology 89/90*, pp. 154–158. Guilford, CT: Dushkin.

Stasio, M. (1989) Between two worlds. In E. Angeloni, ed., *Annual Editions: Anthropology 89/90*, pp. 159–162. Guilford, CT: Dushkin.

Wilber, D. N. (1976) *Iran, Past and Present*. Princeton: Princeton University Press.

NATIVE AMERICANS

Adair, J., and K. W. Deuschle. (1970) *The People's Health*. New York: Appleton-Century-Crofts.

Bozof, R. P. (1972) Some Navaho attitudes toward available medical care. *American Journal of Public Health* 62: 1620–1624.

Coulehan, J. H. (1980) Navaho Indian medicine: Implications for healing. *Journal of Family Practice* 10: 55–61.

Dajer, T. (1989, July) Medicine man. *Discover,* pp. 47–51.

Dennis, W. (1972) *The Hopi Child.* New York: Arno Press.

Driver, H. E. (1969) *Indians of North America.* Chicago: University of Chicago Press.

Edwards, E. D., and M. E. Edwards. (1980) American Indians: Working with individuals and groups. *Social Casework* 61(8): 498–506.

Jewell, D. P. (1979) A case of a "psychotic" Navaho Indian male. In N. Klein, ed., *Culture, Curers & Contagion,* pp. 155–165. Novato, CA: Chandler & Sharp.

Joe, J., C. Gallerito, and J. Pino. (1976) Cultural health traditions: American Indian perspectives. In M. Branch and P. Paxton, eds., *Providing Safe Nursing Care to Ethnic People of Color,* pp. 81–98. New York: Appleton-Century-Crofts.

Kniep-Hardy, M., and M. A. Burkhardt. (1977) Nursing the Navaho. *American Journal of Nursing* 77, 95–96.

Kuttner, R. E., and A. B. Lorincz. (1967) Alcoholism and addiction in urbanized Sioux Indians. *Mental Hygiene* 51: 530–542.

McNickle, K. (1968, August) The sociocultural setting of Indian life. *American Journal of Psychiatry,* pp. 115–119.

Pratson, F. J. (1970) *Land of the Four Directions.* Old Greenwich, CT: Chatham Press.

Primeaux, M. (1977) Caring for the American Indian patient. *American Journal of Nursing* 77: 91–94.

Primeaux, M., and G. Henderson. (1981) American Indian patient care. In G. Henderson and M. Primeaux, eds., *Transcultural Health Care.* pp. 239–254. Menlo Park, CA: Addison-Wesley.

Stone, E. (1962) *Medicine among the American Indians.* New York: Hafner.

Vogel, V. J. (1981) American Indian medicine. In G. Henderson and M. Primeaux, eds., *Transcultural Health Care,* pp. 239–254. Menlo Park, CA: Addison-Wesley.

Wilson, U. M. (1983) Nursing care of American Indian patients. In M. S. Orque, B. Bloch, and L. S. A. Monrroy, eds., *Ethnic Nursing Care: A Multicultural Approach,* pp. 271–295. St. Louis: C. V. Mosby.

Yukl, T. A., and R. Klein. (1976, August) Thoughts and observations on innovation of an Indian clinic in the emergency ward at Massachusetts General Hospital. *Association of American Indian Physicians,* pp. 10–12.

Special Topics

BIRTH

Affonso, D. D. (1978) The Filipino American. In A. L. Clark, ed., *Culture, Childbearing and Health Professionals.* Philadelphia: F. A. Davis.

Bushnell, J. M. (1981) Northwest Coast American Indians' beliefs about childbirth. *Issues in Health Care of Women* 3(4): 249–261.

Clark, A. L., ed. (1978) *Culture, Childbearing and Health Professionals.* Philadelphia: F. A. Davis.

Darabi, K. F., and V. Ortiz. (1987) Childbearing among young Latino women in the U.S. *American Journal of Public Health* 77(1): 25–28.

Farris, L. S. (1976) Approaches to caring for the American Indian maternity patient. *American Journal of Maternal Child Nursing* 1(2): 82–87.

Gaviria, M., G. Stern, and S. L. Schensul. (1982) Sociocultural factors and perinatal health in a Mexican-American community. *Journal of the National Medical Association* 74(10): 983–989.

Gibbs, C. E., H. W. Martin, and M. Gutierrez. (1974) Patterns of reproductive health care among the poor of San Antonio, Texas. *American Journal of Public Health* 64: 37–40.

Hallmark, G., and M. Findlay. (1982) Cesarean birth in the operating room. *AORN Journal* 36: 978–984.

Holck, S. E., C. W. Warren, L. Morris, and R. W. Rochat. (1982) Need for family planning services among Anglo and Hispanic women in U.S. counties bordering Mexico. *Family Planning Perspectives* 14(3): 155–159.

Hollingsworth, A., L. Brown, and D. Broaten. (1980) The refugees and child-bearing: What to expect. *RN Magazine* 43: 45–48.

Hook, E. B. (1978) Dietary cravings and aversions during pregnancy. *American Journal of Clinical Nutrition* 31: 1355–1362.

Horn, B. M. (1981) Cultural concepts and postpartal care. *Nursing and Health Care* 2(9): 516–517, 526–527.

Jimenez, M. H., and N. Newton. (1979) Activity and work during pregnancy and the postpartum period: A cross-cultural study of 202 societies. *American Journal of Obstetrics and Gynecology* 135(2): 171–176.

Johnston, M. (1980) Cultural variations in professional and parenting patterns. *JOGN Nursing* 9: 9–13.

Jordan, B. (1978) The cross-cultural comparison of birthing systems: Towards a biosocial analysis. In B. Jordan, ed., *Birth in Four Cultures*, pp. 32–65. St. Albans, VT: Eden Press Women's Publications.

Kay, M. A., ed. (1982) *Anthropology of Human Birth*. Philadelphia: F. A. Davis.

Kitzinger, S. (1977) Challenges in antenatal education. *Nursing Mirror* 144: 19–22.

Mead, M., and N. Newton. (1967) Cultural patterning of perinatal behavior. In S. A. Richardson and A. F. Guttmacher, eds., *Childbearing: Its Social and Psychological Aspects*, pp. 142–243. Baltimore: Williams & Wilkins.

Meleis, A. I., and L. Sorrell. (1981) Bridging cultures: Arab American women and their birth experiences. *Maternal Child Nursing* 6: 171–176.

Minkler, D. H. (1983) The role of a community-based satellite clinic in the perinatal care of non-English speaking immigrants. *Western Journal of Medicine* 139: 905–909.

Pillsbury, B. (1982) "Doing the month": Confinement and convalescence of Chinese women after childbirth. In M. A. Kay, ed., *Anthropology of Human Birth*, pp. 119–146. Philadelphia: F. A. Davis.

Wertz, R. W., and D. C. Wertz. (1977) *Lying In: A History of Childbirth in America*. New York: Macmillan.

Williams, M. A. (1976) Ethnocultural responses to hysterectomy: Implications for nursing. In P. J. Brink, ed., *Transcultural Nursing*, pp. 219–233. Englewood Cliffs, NJ: Prentice-Hall.

Williams, R. L., N. J. Benkin, and E. J. Clingman. (1986) Pregnancy outcomes among Spanish-surname women in California. *American Journal of Public Health* 76(4): 387–391.

Zapeda, M. (1982) Selected maternal-infant care practices of Spanish-speaking women. *JOGN Nursing* 11(6): 371–374.

DEATH AND DYING

DeSpelder, L., and A. Strickland. (1987) *The Last Dance: Encountering Death & Dying.* 2d ed. Mountain View, CA: Mayfield.
French, J., and D. Schwartz. (1976) Terminal care at home in two cultures. In P. Brink, ed., *Transcultural Nursing,* pp. 247–255. Englewood Cliffs, NJ: Prentice-Hall.
Kalish, R. A., and D. K. Reynolds. (1981) *Death and Ethnicity: A Psychocultural Study.* Amityville, NY: Baywood Press.
Lally, M. M. (1978) Last rites and funeral customs of minority groups. *Midwife Health Visitor and Community Nurse* 14: 224–225.
Rosenblatt, P., R. Walsh, and D. Jackson. (1976) *Grief and Mourning in Cross-Cultural Perspective.* New Haven, CT: HRAF Press.
Ross, H. M. (1981) Societal/cultural views regarding death and dying. *Topics in Clinical Nursing* 3(3): 1–16.
Shibles, W. (1974) *Death: An Interdisciplinary Analysis.* Whitewater, WI: Language Press.
Walker, C. (1982) Attitudes to death and bereavement among cultural minority groups. *Nursing Times* (December 15): 2106–2109.

DIET

Crane, N. T. (1983) Nutritional status of Hispanic Americans. *Public Health Currents* 23(5): 4–7.
Friemer, N., D. Echenberg, and N. Kretchmer. (1983) Cultural variation: Nutritional and clinical implications. *Western Journal of Medicine* 139(6): 928–933.
Gonzales, N. (1966) Filipino culture and food habits. *Philippine Journal of Nutrition* 19: 194–201.
Hook, E. B. (1978) Dietary cravings and aversions during pregnancy. *American Journal of Clinical Nutrition* 31: 1355–1362.
Ludman, E. K., and J. M. Newman. (1984) Yin and yang in the health-related food practices of three Chinese groups. *Journal of Nutrition Education* 16: 3–7.
Payne, Z. A. (1980) Diet and folk remedies: The influence of cultural patterns on medical management. *Urban Health* 9: 24–28.
Tong, A. (1986) Food habits of Vietnamese immigrants. *Family Economics Review* 2: 28–30.
Whang, J. (1981) Chinese traditional food therapy. *Journal of the American Dietetic Association* 78: 55–57.

FEMALE CIRCUMCISION

Davies, N. (1984) *The Rampant God.* New York: William Morrow.
El Dareer, A. (1982) *Woman, Why Do You Weep?* London: Zed.

Harden, B. (1985, July 29) Female circumcision: Painful, risky, and little girls beg for it. *Washington Post,* pp. 15–16.

Lightfoot-Klein, H. (1990) *Prisoners of Ritual.* Binghamton, NY: Haworth Press.

Romberg, R. (1985) *Circumcision: The Painful Dilemma.* South Hadley, MA: Bergin & Garvey.

Shaw, E. (1985) Female circumcision. *American Journal of Nursing* 85(6): 684–687.

Verzin, J. A. (1975, October) Sequelae of female circumcision. *Tropical Doctor,* pp. 163–169.

FOLK MEDICINE

Currier, R. L. (1966) The hot-cold syndrome and symbolic balance in Mexican and Spanish-American folk medicine. *Ethnology* 5: 251–263.

Delgado, M. (1979) Herbal medicine in the Puerto Rican community. *Health in Social Work* 4: 24–40.

Edgerton, R. B., M. Karno, and I. Fernandez. (1970) Curanderismo in the metropolis. *American Journal of Psychotherapy* 24(1): 124–134.

Garrison, V. (1977) Doctor, "espiritista" or psychiatrist?: Health seeking behavior in a Puerto Rican neighborhood of New York City. *Medical Anthropology* 1(2): 65–180.

Hook, E. B. (1978) Dietary cravings and aversions during pregnancy. *American Journal of Clinical Nutrition* 31: 1355–1362.

Jordan, W. C. (1979) The roots and practices of voodoo medicine in America. *Urban Health* 8: 38–41.

Kaptchuk, T. J. (1983) *The Web That Has No Weaver: Understanding Chinese Medicine.* New York: Congdon & Weed.

Kelly, I. (1965) *Folk Practice in North Mexico: Birth Customs, Folk Medicine and Spiritualism in the Laguna Zone.* Austin: University of Texas Press.

Kiev, A. (1968) *Curanderismo: Mexican-American Folk Psychiatry.* New York: Free Press.

Lichstein, P. R. (1982) Can a physician heal a 'hex'? *Hospital Practice* (November): 125–132.

Maduro, R. (1983) Curanderismo and Latino views of disease and curing. *Western Journal of Medicine* 139: 868–874.

Martin, M. (1981) Native American medicine: Thoughts for post-traditional healers. *Journal of the American Medical Association* 245: 141–143.

Martinez, C., and H. W. Martinez. (1966) Folk disease among urban Mexican-Americans. *Journal of the American Medical Association* 196: 161–164.

McKenzie, J. L., and N. J. Chrisman. (1977) Healing herbs, gods, and magic: Folk health beliefs among Filipino-Americans. *Nursing Outlook* 25: 326–329.

McNall, M. (1989) Dialogue with excellence: Healing we cannot explain. *American Journal of Nursing* 89(9): 1162–1163.

Messer, E. (1981) Hot-cold classification: Theoretical and practical implications of a Mexican study. *Social Science Medicine* 15B: 133–145.

Muecke, M. A. (1983) In search of healers: Southeast Asian refugees in the American health care system. *Western Journal of Medicine* 129: 835–840.

Payne, Z. A. (1980) Diet and folk remedies: The influence of cultural patterns on medical management. *Urban Health* 9: 24–28.

Press, I. (1971) The urban curandero. *American Anthropologist* 73: 741–756.

Sandler, A. P., and L. S. Chan. (1978) Mexican-American folk belief in a pediatric emergency room. *Medical Care* 16: 778–784.

Saunders, L., and G. W. Hewes. (1953) Folk medicine and medical practice. *Journal of Medical Education* 28: 43–46.

Searle, C. (1980) The power of the folk healer. *Nursing Mirror* (December 4): 30–34.

Snow, L. F. (1974) Folk medical beliefs and their implications for the care of patients: A review based on studies among Black Americans. *Annals of Internal Medicine* 81: 82–96.

Snow, L. F. (1979) Voodoo illness in the Black population. In N. Klein, ed., *Culture, Curers & Contagion*, pp. 179–184. Novato, CA: Chandler & Sharp.

Stewart, H. (1971) Kindling of hope in the disadvantaged: A study of the Afro-American healer. *Mental Hygiene* 55: 96–100.

Tinling, D. C. (1967) Voodoo, root work, and medicine. *Psychosomatic Medicine* 29: 483–490.

Toohey, J. V. (1980) Curanderas and brujas: Herbal healing in a Mexican American community. *Health Education* 11: 2–4.

Torrey, E. F. (1986) *Witchdoctors and Psychiatrists.* New York: Harper & Row.

Trotter, R. T. (1981) Remedios caseros: Mexican-American home remedies and community health problems. *Social Science Medicine* 15B: 107–114.

Weimer, S. R., and N. L. Mintz. (1976–77) Health practice at the technologic/folk interface: Witchcraft as a culture-specific diagnosis. *International Journal of Psychiatry & Medicine* 1: 351–362.

Yeatman, G. W. (1980) *Cao gio* (coin rubbing): Vietnamese attitudes toward health care. *Journal of the American Medical Association* 244: 2748–2749.

PAIN

Baer, E., L. J. Davitz, and R. Lieb. (1970) Inferences of physical pain and psychological distress in relation to verbal and nonverbal patient communication. *Nursing Research* 19: 28–34, 42.

Davitz, L. J., Y. Sameshima, and J. Davitz. (1976) Suffering as viewed in six different cultures. *American Journal of Nursing* 76: 1296.

Martinelli, A. M. (1987) Pain and ethnicity. *AORN Journal* 46(2): 273–281.

McMahon, M. A., and P. Miller. (1978) Pain response: The influence of psychosocial-cultural factors. *Nursing Forum* 17(1): 58.

Reizian, A. and A. I. Meleis. (1986) Arab-Americans' perceptions of and responses to pain. *Critical Care Nurse* 6(6): 30–37.

Wolff, H. G., and S. Langley. (1975) Cultural factors and the response to pain. In M. Weisenberg, ed., *Pain: Clinical and Experimental Perspectives*, pp. 144–151. St. Louis: C. V. Mosby.

Zborowski, M. (1952) Cultural components in response to pain. *Journal of Social Issues* 8: 16–30.

Zola, I. K. (1966) Culture and symptoms: An analysis of patients' presenting complaints. *American Sociological Review* 31: 615–630.

RELIGION

Ausubel, N. (1964) *The Book of Jewish Knowledge.* New York: Crown.

Backman, M. V. (1983) *Christian Churches of America.* New York: Scribner's.

Berkowitz, P., and N. S. Berkowitz. (1967) The Jewish patient in the hospital. *American Journal of Nursing* 67: 2335–2337.

Christian Science Publishing Society. (1974) *Questions and Answers on Christian Science.* Boston: Christian Science.

Donin, H. H. (1972) *To Be a Jew.* New York: Basic Books.

Guttmacher, S. and J. Elinson. (1971) Ethno-religious variations in perceptions of illness. *Social Science Medicine* 5: 117–125.

Haneef, S. (1979) *What Everyone Should Know about Islam and Muslims.* Chicago: Kazi.

Kahn, M. Z. (1964) *Islam: Its Meaning for Modern Man.* London: Routledge & Kegan Paul.

Kinsley, D. R. (1982) *Hinduism.* Englewood Cliffs, NJ: Prentice-Hall.

Lippman, T. W. (1982) *Understanding Islam.* New York: New American Library.

Luce, M. R., ed. (1957) *The World's Great Religions.* New York: Time.

McConkie, B. R. (1979) *Mormon Doctrine.* Salt Lake City: Bookcraft.

Mishr, R. P. (1982) *Hinduism: The Faith of the Future.* Princeton, NJ: Humanities Press.

Prager, D., and J. Telushkin. (1981) *The Nine Questions People Ask about Judaism.* New York: Simon and Schuster.

Rockowitz, R. J., J. W. Korpela, and K. C. Hunter. (1981) Social work dilemma: When religion and medicine clash. *Health and Social Work* 6: 5–11.

Rosten, L., ed. (1975) *Religions of America.* New York: Simon and Schuster.

Rozovsky, L. E. (1971) Blood (Part I): Jehovah's Witnesses and the law. *Canadian Hospital* 48: 41–42.

Wheat, M. E., H. Brownstein, and V. Kvitash. (1983) Aspects of medical care of Soviet Jewish emigrés. *Western Journal of Medicine* 139: 900–904.

Yoshinori, T. (1983) *The Heart of Buddhism.* New York: Crossroad.

VALUES

Arensberg, C. M., and A. H. Niehoff. (1971) American cultural values. In L. Holmes, ed., *Readings in General Anthropology*, pp. 303–314. New York: Ronald Press.

Kluckhohn, F. (1976) Dominant and variant value orientations. In P. Brink, ed., *Transcultural Nursing. A Book of Readings*, pp. 63–81. Englewood Cliffs, NJ: Prentice-Hall.

Oring, E. (1979) From uretics to uremics: A contribution toward the ethnography of peeing. In N. Klein, ed., *Culture, Curers & Contagion*, pp. 15–21. Novato, CA: Chandler & Sharp.

MISCELLANEOUS

Cannon, W. B. (1965) Voodoo death. In W. A. Lessa and E. Z. Vogt, eds., *Reader in Comparative Religion*, pp. 321–327. New York: Harper & Row.

Clements, F. E. (1932) Primitive concepts of disease. *University of California Publications in American Archeology and Ethnology* 32: 185–252.

Daughtry, C. (1981) An ecologic perspective of child abuse. In C. Getty and W. Humphreys, eds., *Understanding the Family*, pp. 298–331. New York: Appleton-Century-Crofts.

Evans-Pritchard, E. E. (1976) *Witchcraft, Oracles, and Magic among the Azande.* Oxford: Clarendon Press.

Harris, M. (1974) *Cows, Pigs, Wars and Witches.* New York: Vintage Books.

Kennedy, J. G. (1967) Nubian Zar ceremonies as psychotherapy. *Human Organization* 4: 185–194.

Levine, R., and D. Campbell. (1972) *Ethnocentrism: Theories of Conflict, Ethnic Attitudes, and Group Behavior.* New York: John Wiley.

Lewis, O. (1966) The culture of poverty. *Scientific American* 215(4): 19–25.

Maloney, C., ed. (1976) *The Evil Eye.* New York: Columbia University Press.

Nguyen, A. (1980) *Chinese Astrology.* New York: Arbor.

Reminick, R. A. (1977) The evil eye belief among the Amhara of Ethiopia. In D. Landy, ed., *Culture, Disease, and Healing,* pp. 218–226. New York: Macmillan.

Subject Index

Note: Numbers refer to case studies, not pages. They correspond to numbers found on the outside margins of the text, àt the beginning of each case study.

Body Image
Fat: 134
Hair: 87, 130, 131, 132
  Pubic: 87
Scars: 132

Communication:
9, 10, 11, 110, 111
Eye contact: 2, 68
Gestures: 13
Idioms: 3, 4, 5, 6, 7
Insults: 5, 6, 7, 13
Interpreters: 1, 9, 38
Language: 6, 7, 10, 11, 12
Names: 8
Pronouns: 12

Diet:
42, 43, 44, 45, 46, 97, 99, 103, 125
Dates: 43
Food: 36, 42, 43, 45, 46, 97, 99
Kosher: 44
Meat with dairy: 44
Pork: 42, 44
Shellfish: 44

Disease Etiology
Body balance: 45, 46, 98, 99, 100, 120, 121
  Hot-cold: 45, 46, 98, 99, 100, 120, 121, 122
  Yin-yang: 46, 121

Breach of taboo: 31, 131
  Sin: 31
Food deprivation: 43
Supernatural: 39, 47, 48, 126
  Evil eye: 39
  Hex: 48
  Red: 40
  Voodoo: 126
  Witchcraft: 47, 48

Ethnic Groups
Armenian: 120
Asian: 3, 4, 5, 9, 10, 11, 12, 13, 18, 19, 20, 23, 29, 35, 46, 49, 50, 54, 55, 56, 57, 61, 63, 65, 74, 75, 76, 78, 79, 85, 90, 97, 98, 99, 100, 102, 115, 117, 118, 119, 121, 129, 135
  Cambodian: 115, 128
  Chinese: 3, 11, 18, 20, 46, 55, 78, 79, 97, 117, 129
  Filipino: 5, 9, 13, 19, 29, 35, 54, 75, 76, 90, 100
  Japanese: 12, 49, 56, 61, 77, 121, 129
  Korean: 4, 63, 65, 74, 118, 135
  Laotian: 23, 57
  Taiwanese: 78
  Vietnamese: 50, 85, 98, 99, 102, 119
Black: 6, 7, 8, 17, 26, 28, 31, 64, 73, 88, 89, 90, 114, 125, 126, 133
  African: 17, 26, 73, 89, 133
  American: 6, 7, 8, 28, 31, 64, 88, 90, 114, 124, 125, 126

This book was set in Baskerville and Eras typefaces. Baskerville was designed by John Baskerville at his private press in Birmingham, England, in the eighteenth century. The first typeface to depart from oldstyle typeface design, Baskerville has more variation between thick and thin strokes. In an effort to insure that the thick and thin strokes of his typeface reproduced well on paper, John Baskerville developed the first wove paper, the surface of which was much smoother than the laid paper of the time. The development of wove paper was partly responsible for the introduction of typefaces classified as modern, which have even more contrast between thick and thin strokes.

Eras was designed in 1969 by Studio Hollenstein in Paris for the Wagner Typefoundry. A contemporary script-like version of a sans-serif typeface, the letters of Eras have a monotone stroke and are slightly inclined.

Printed on acid-free paper.